The ABC's of Stress

The ABC's of Stress

A SUBMARINE PSYCHOLOGIST'S PERSPECTIVE

Benjamin B. Weybrew

Foreword by Edward L. Beach

PRAEGER

Westport, Connecticut
London

Library of Congress Cataloging-in-Publication Data

Weybrew, Benjamin B.
The ABC's of stress : a submarine psychologist's perspective /
Benjamin B. Weybrew ; foreword by Edward L. Beach.
p. cm.
Includes bibliographical references and index.
ISBN 0-275-94233-3 (alk. paper)
1. Submarine medicine. 2. Stress (Psychology). I. Title.
[DNLM: 1. Stress, Psychological. 2. Submarine Medicine. WD 650
W546a]
RC1005.W49 1992
155.9'63—dc20
DNLM/DLC 92-11956

British Library Cataloguing in Publication Data is available.

Library of Congress Catalog Card Number: 92-11956
ISBN: 0-275-94233-3

First published in 1992

Praeger Publishers, 88 Post Road West, Westport, CT 06881
An imprint of Greenwood Publishing Group, Inc.

Printed in the United States of America

The paper used in this book complies with the
Permanent Paper Standard issued by the National
Information Standards Organization (Z39.48-1984).

10 9 8 7 6 5 4 3 2 1

To my wife, Betzy, a constant among variables,
and to our son, Dana, and his wonderful family,
his wife, Teresa, and their two children, Lauren and Adam.
With love to all.

El tensio, sic vis. (As the stretching, so is the force).

—Sir Robert Hooke,
a seventeenth-century English physicist

Contents

Figures and Tables

FIGURES

TABLES

Foreword

It is perhaps no surprise to Ben Weybrew, my shipmate in USS *Triton* during our submerged, world circumnavigation, that I've secretly been waiting for this book—at least for some detailed treatment of the subject—for quite some time. That voyage, I honestly think, made me into something of an amateur psychologist, but in the event of need, Dr. Benjamin Weybrew, a practicing psychologist put aboard at the last minute to study *us*, was available. He found many willing subjects for his ongoing study and more than once reassured me that, from his view, everything was just fine.

As a World War II submariner, I'm one of a remaining few who have experienced stress to the ultimate degree: submerged under enemy attack and with little power to help oneself. World War II submariners, accustomed to cruising in the highest possible state of alert, ready instantly to dive out from under an attacking aircraft, or slam into battle stations without preparatory notice and go on the attack—or conversely, to gird for depth charging, go deep, lie silent, and pray the explosions don't get too close—were prime targets for the study of physical and mental stress. Often we wondered if anyone else in the whole world had any idea of what it was really like. We were pretty one-sided then, but under the circumstances, we had a point. The unwritten rules of submarine combat put maximum pressure on everyone. Surprisingly, there were few crack ups.

After the war, there was a terrific letdown but also more time to think. Among the thoughts that occurred to me was the appreciation that, for many involved reasons, those years of stress were actually enjoyable—not entirely, of course, but in their summation (since I survived). The stresses among submariners now, in peacetime, are very different, but they are still powerful, possessing an entirely new dimension because of nuclear power and our consequent greatly expanded capabilities. I was one of the fortunate few able to shift from the old directly into the new, and the privilege of commanding the nuclear submarine *Triton* on her shakedown cruise as she went, fully submerged, around the world was arguably the culmination of my naval career.

There was stress during the *Triton's* cruise—a great deal of it—beginning before we ever left port, but it was distinctly different from anything anyone assigned to the ship had ever felt. First there was the preparation phase, all to be done in total secrecy and with no time whatever to spare: ten days of strenuous work to provision the ship, obtain three times our regular allowance of navigational charts, plan for personal as well as medical emergencies of all kinds and for families left at home, get aboard all possible spare parts—and some that were not on our allowance list but that we thought we might need anyway (fighting the bureaucracy on *that* one was special all the way). Under the burden of secrecy, we had to make up our own rules, get what we needed, and do what we had to do, without giving away the game. There was simply no time to argue the fine points.

Once under way, with a crew that had not yet been informed what they were about, everything was totally different. Now the problem was to keep the crew on their toes, maintain a high level of activity, avoid boredom, and keep things on a high plane of motivation. All this, of course, comes under the heading of morale, and well I knew the old naval adage that the ultimate morale officer is the captain. Early on, I realized that what this particular crew needed from me was not pressure but the light touch. Once informed of our objective, their enthusiasm infected everything they did, and here or there might easily have caused stress-related dysfunction. Extended separation from home and family with no means of communication was not a problem—submariners are used to that—but bearing down too much on the job might be. Not a man aboard was not doing his utmost to make the voyage a success. My concern was about our performance in an emergency, being at the same time unable to predict what emergencies might be in store for us. It was important, I thought, to hold back on the pressure until a really tough problem came up. This happened several times, as I knew it would, and I was glad I had something in reserve.

Things went pretty well all in all. We handled all our emergencies in stride, and I think Dr. Weybrew will bear me out. All the same, everyone in the ship was fully occupied during that cruise, especially me, and many times since I've wished I had made more time to talk with him as we went along.

Now Dr. Ben has synthesized his observations over a lifetime of study of American submariners, and everyone will profit. Despite some media "hype," we are not all that different from normal average people, but we do have a wonderful instrument that few truly appreciate, and we do know how to use it. *Triton* was one of the early nuclear subs, and at the time of our circumnavigation we established a record for distance and time submerged that stood for many years. For all I know, it stands yet, although anytime one of today's submarines needs to do better, it will simply go off and do it as a matter of ordinary business.

The submarines and their weapons of today are so vastly superior to what we had only a few years ago that to us old-timers the comparison is scary, but there is one thing that hasn't changed: the make-up of the human beings who are the masters of these things. It's high time we learned more about them and how they are likely to perform under various conditions. So far, it's been done by intuitive judgment, and some commanders are better at it than others. Scientific study cannot but add to the ability of all of us to handle the intangibles we've dealt with empirically all these years, and that's what Ben Weybrew, and this book, are all about.

Edward L. Beach
Captain, USN (Ret.)

Preface

There was no hesitancy in selecting the title for this book. We need to get back to basic principles, the ABC's, in the ever-expanding field of *stress*. Since World War II, professional publications of stress-related topics by physicians, physiologists, psychologists, sociologists, and other behaviorally and medically oriented scientists have appeared in increasing numbers year by year. The focus of these papers has been upon theories of stress, upon the identification of variables associated with stress, and upon approaches to the development of effective stress management strategies.

As we enter the last decade of the twentieth century, stress-related issues have become the "wastebasket category," a scapegoat for a wide range of undiagnosed illnesses, such as breathing, skin, and intestinal disorders—even cancer[44]. Stress has also been blamed for a number of military catastrophes. For example, an article from the *New York Times* News Service (dated August 3, 1988) summarized the findings of the panel investigating the deaths of 290 civilians resulting from a missile attack by the U.S. Navy cruiser *Vincennes* on an Iranian commercial jet in the Persian Gulf. The screaming headline read, "Stress cited in downing of jet." Further into the piece, the statement was made flatly, "crew error arising from the psychological stress of being in combat for the first time was responsible for the disaster." In the same edition, an Associated Press article summarizing a psychiatric study of Vietnam veterans carried the lead sentence: "one out of seven Vietnam veterans suffers from Post-traumatic Stress Syndrome." Finally, demonstrating the broad public concern about the real or presumed debilitating effects of *stress* was the publication in 1988 of the *The Jobs Rated Almanac*, which contains ratings of 250 jobs in terms of their capacity to induce stress. After three decades, stress still remains a prime research subject, as attested by the intensity of the in-house arguments that have been and are still being waged over issues dealing with the conceptualization of terms and selection of research strategies in this complex field[30, 67].

The immediate impetus for writing this book arose from the observation that the number, but not necessarily the quality, of lay-level, stress-related articles and books appearing in bookstores and magazine shops was increasing rapidly. So, why add another book on the subject of stress to this literary clutter? The answer is straightforward. The reading public quite simply has become confused as to what the term *stress* has as a referent: to stimulus conditions, to patterns of response to these conditions, or to an interaction between stimulus and response. *The ABC's of Stress* focuses on the identification of specific referents for the stress-related terms being used, on the specification of the variable interactions constituting the causes of stress, and finally on practical, and to an extent, empirically based recommendations for the alleviation and control of the debilitating effects of stress.

Last, the magnitude of the stress problem, economically speaking, is overwhelming. For example, assuming, as many medical experts do, that stress contributes significantly to heart disease, something on the order of 60 billion lost workdays at a cost of $30 billion occur annually in the United States because of heart attacks alone. These facts translate to the betting odds that at least one out of five men in the work force will suffer a fatal or debilitative heart attack before they reach retirement age[52].

ACKNOWLEDGMENTS

I am grateful to three outstanding psychologists, all of whom are deceased. These renowned scientists greatly influenced my theoretical orientation on the topic of stress during and after my doctoral training—Karl Muenzinger, a field theorist, University of Colorado; Marion Wenger, a psychophysiologist, University of California at Los Angeles; and Walter Miles, a true electicist, U.S. Naval Submarine Medical Research Laboratory, New London, Connecticut. All of these prolific researchers exposed me to a plethora of ideas pertaining to the topic of stress, ideas that I am only now beginning to sort out after more than three decades. Walter Miles especially taught me the real meaning of the word "science."

Also, my thanks to some half-dozen commanding officers and their staffs of the Submarine Medical Research Laboratory, where I had the good fortune to be employed from 1952 until my retirement in 1979. These submarine medical officers were responsible for clearing the bureaucratic impediments, so that my staff and I were able to collect a variety of data related to nuclear submariners' reactions to the unique stressors of submerged missions, often exceeding eighty days' duration. Most of the data and many of the inferences therefrom contained in this book originated from this source.

Finally, as a member of the faculty of the University of New Haven, Connecticut, I am indebted to the nearly 200 graduate students who participated in my seminars on stress during the past eleven years. I especially wish to express my appreciation to two of my recent graduate students: Carol Lozanov-Miccio for a comprehensive review of the literature dealing with the relationship between exercise physiology and stress, and Ann-Marie Dombroski for a similar review on the relationship between nutrition and stress. Selected research findings from both of these excellent reviews are included in Chapter 8 of this text. All of these highly motivated students tenaciously forced me to operationally define each and every stress-related term I used in these seminars.

I
Overview

The word "stress" is apparently derived from the Latin verb *stringere*, meaning to tighten up[108]. In the 1930's, Walter Cannon used the expression "critical stress levels" to refer to environmental conditions that resulted in the disruption of states of biological equilibrium or homeostasis[21]. In the 1950's, Hans Selye, sometimes called the father of stress, used the term stress in his monumental text to refer to the internal biochemical states resulting from acute or chronic exposure to environmental irritants or "stressors." Summarized succinctly in reference[56], at least eight models or mini-theories of stress have appeared in the literature since Selye's early publications[106]. The focus of these models ranges from perception of environmental events, psychosomatic tension, and the physiological processes underlying stress to the cognitive processes and the social milieu associated with stress-related conditions[26].

PHILOSOPHICAL POSITIONS RELATED TO STRESS

Stress theorists attempting to explain the causes, mechanisms, and control strategies of stress have tended to assume the validity of one or another of two philosophical models: the medical or diseasism model or the behavioral or psychological model. These two models are compared below.

Diseasism or Medical Model	Behavioral or Psychological Model
a. Distributions of stress-related symptoms are dichotomous (i.e., stressed vs. nonstressed).	a. Distributions are continuous.
b. POSR (Patterns of Stress Reactivity) are processes different in *kind*.	b. POSR are processes different in *degree*.

c. Concern is for what a person *has* (i.e., like catching the flu).	c. Concern is for what a person *Does* and *Feels*.
d. POSR results from predispositional factors, organ deficiencies, bad genes.	d. POSR results from predispositional factors interacting with learned maladaptive life-styles.
e. POSR caused by a localizable defect, a pathogen.	e. POSR results from maladaptive life-styles.
f. Results in stereotyping, ignoring individual differences and environmental influences.	f. The focus is on individual differences in the context of environmental influences.
g. Assumes every stress reaction has a specific, identifiable cause.	g. Assumes POSR have a multiplicity of interacting causes.
h. Rumpelstiltskin Fallacy holds (*see* Glossary).	h. Does not hold, in fact, may be counterproductive.
i. "Alcoholism" as an example of contracting a stress-related disease, which, if criminal behavior ensues, may result in jail time—for getting sick?	i. "Alcoholic abuse" as an example of a maladaptive reactive pattern to a stressful environment.

The medical model, consisting of a dichotomization of the disease continuum, is a modernization of the ancient conceptual approach of stereotyping objects, including people, into mutually exclusive categories. For example, Hippocrates (c. Third Century B.C.) proposed a classification system for people consisting of four types coinciding with the so-called body humors: excessive yellow bile-choleric (irritable), excessive black bile-melancholic (depressed), excessive blood-sanguine (optimistic), and excessive phlegmatic (listless). In the early twentieth century, the Swiss psychiatrist Carl Jung categorized persons into two classes: extroverts, emotions expressed outwardly, and introverts, emotions expressed inwardly[3]. Finally, a late twentieth-century extrapolation of Jung's dual typology was the twofold classification of disparate personal life-styles into Type A and Type B personalities. In this system, Type A personalities are characterized by a restive, time-constrained, competitive, and hostile life-style underpinned by well-established, unwavering beliefs and attitudes that they must excel in all areas and must develop their potential to its fullest. In contrast, Type B personalities, although as strongly motivated as Type As, tend to adopt a more relaxed, unhurried, affable and noncompetitive life-style, with more realistic attitudes supporting life goals derived from a practical appraisal of the possibilities afforded by the environment.

Enter stress theorists. Although the empirical evidence is equivocal, it has been and continues to be argued that persons typifying the Type A trait pattern may experience higher levels of stress than Type Bs and, either as a concomitant or a consequence of stress, are more likely to develop coronary heart disease later on in life[40]. Following from this long history of the practice of health care professionals to categorize disease entities and personality trait patterns into "types" is the present practice of classifying stress reactions into diagnostic categories. A modern example of this practice is PTSD (Post-traumatic Stress Disorder) applied to certain disturbed veterans of the Vietnam campaign[29].

The practice of typing or classifying personalities or disease states into mutually exclusive categories, however, results in the omission of two important kinds of data necessary for understanding stress. First, this approach tends to omit data pertaining to individual differences within a given type, Type A and Type B, for example. Second, this practice also omits the interactive effects of the environment in which the "typed" behavior or disease process occurs or develops. The so-called class theoretical fallacy described by the ancient Greek philosophers makes essentially the same point. That is, because a person belongs to a specific class or set (Type A or B, Jew or Gentile, black or white race, Catholic or Protestant, etc.) does not mean that those included within this class are identical. Indeed, individual differences within type or set are often considerable. The part that this fallacy plays in the establishment and maintenance of social prejudices, bigotry and narrow-mindedness, and, for that matter, the diseasism model of stress-related illnesses, should be obvious.

This book contains partial solutions to the problem of the omission of these kinds of data, the result being a more integrated approach to the topic of stress, incorporating selected aspects of both the medical and psychological models. The net result is a significant enhancement of the fund of knowledge relating to the dynamics of stress and stress-related conditions.

NEW PERSPECTIVES FOR THE STUDY OF STRESS

We begin with Kurt Lewin's often-cited equation: $B = f(P \times E)$, where f = function of, B = behavior, P = personality, and E = environment. A simple verbalization of this equation might be: An individual's behavior depends upon the interaction of the characteristics of that person with selected aspects of the environment. It is seen that Lewin's equation includes the two sources of data omitted in the typology approach, namely, individual personality differences and environmental influences[70].

In a sense, this book is an extrapolation and clarification of this equation. Chapter 2 presents an extension of Lewin's concept of motives as vectors, having both force and directionality. Emotions and conflict are also explained in vector terminology. Chapter 3 presents the ABC model of stress, in which the directional characteristics of motives are explained by the relationship of the "Need Prepotency Profile" to the "A" (of ABC's) for *antecedent* conditions, to the "B" for the goal-directed *behavior*, and to the "C" for the *consequences* of the goal-directed behavior. Chapter 3 also presents a detailed description of the six major classes of psychophysiological processes constituting stress reactions, or, for the purpose of this book, POSR.

Chapter 4 introduces three discursive equations that expand and clarify Lewin's "personality" (P) and "environmental" (E) interaction in three ways: (a) by describing the mechanism by which the "P" and "E" interrelationship contributes to stress, (b) by providing a practical method for estimating the intensity of the environmental effects, and (c) by identifying the perceptual, motivational, and emotional aspects of personality that contribute to POSR.

Chapter 5 contains a summary of the major classes of environmental stressors, the "E" in Lewin's equation. In addition, this summary includes an estimate of the SEP (Stress Evocation Potential) for each class of stressor, an estimate of the relative accessibility of the means to overcome or adapt to each stressor class, and the time span in a person's life during which the SEP of each stressor category is maximum.

Chapter 6 assumes a worst case scenario, namely, that a person may either be exposed to one or more high-SEP stressor(s) for a relatively brief time or to a low-SEP stressor(s) for a long period of time. In either case, the changes in attitudes and the occurrence of several patterns of psychophysiological and medical symptoms, as well as other possible consequences of elevated POSR, are presented and briefly discussed. Modern, diagnostic categories for these stress-related syndromes are also described.

Chapter 7 asks the question: What kinds of data (biographical, medical, psychophysiological, psychosocial) are the most valid predictors of individual differences in a person's SCC (Stress Coping Capacity)? Examples of the kinds of psychometric instruments used by the U.S. Naval Submarine Service for this predictive function are presented.

The dual problem of both the prevention and treatment of debilitating, sometimes pathological, stress reactions is addressed in Chapter 8. To focus these interrelated problems, two kinds of information are needed. First, an assessment of a person's SCC is needed. This topic was described in Chapter 7. Second, and equally important, is the estimation of the intensity of the stressors being imposed upon a person at a given time. This approximation, called IED (Intensity of Environmental Demands), is approached methodologically by SIRO (Stressor Identification and Rank Ordering), a stressor ranking technique developed and field tested for the submarine service.

Chapter 9 answers three methodological questions central to research in the area of stress. First, *what* kinds of data need to be collected? Second, *how*, by what methodology, should these data be analyzed in order to shed the most light on the major processes involved in POSR? Third, *how*, by what methodological approach(es), can the diverse kinds of stress data be integrated into a model or models explaining the dynamics of stress reactivity?

Finally, Chapter 10, using considerable hyperbole yet adhering closely to the implications of the ABC model of stress, addresses some of the most critical social, geopolitical and cultural issues of our time. Accordingly, the ABC model is applied to the part stress plays in causing the educational deficiencies in the United States, to the subject of the impediments to creativity caused by stress, to the relationship of stress to leadership behavior, to the contribution of stress to the current drug abuse problem, and, finally, to the role of stress in causing and preventing wars.

Following the body of the text is a glossary of 88 stress-related terms and acronyms for the convenience of the reader, and a carefully selected list of 162 references. Also included in the Appendixes are nine experimental tests developed for the U.S. Naval Submarine Service to measure individual differences in the SCC of nuclear submariners. Finally, the appendix also contains an analytical form used to evaluate research proposals dealing with stress-related topics.

In summary, the ABC model of stress is eclectic, incorporating some aspects of certain philosophical viewpoints as well as elements of both the medical and behavioral models. "ABC" is based upon selected principles of the physics of energy, upon modern behavioral reinforcement theory, and upon the computer-age systems concept as applied to stress-related processes.

This book is not meant to be a factually documented text in all instances; in fact, it contains a number of hypotheses pertaining to interactions of stress-related variables for which there often are minimal empirical underpinnings. These "educated guesses" are presented nonetheless for heuristic purposes. Although literature containing a great deal of factual data, originating mainly from nuclear submarine research, is cited, the overriding intent of this book is rather to present a new and different approach to understanding the dynamics of stress by means of the ABC model.

In short, the ABC model of stress has an applied focus for the layperson wishing to enhance his or her stress coping capacity, a theoretical as well as an applied focus for the facilitator in stress management seminars, and a purely theoretical focus for the scientist seeking a new research approach in this ever-expanding area.

2
Theoretical Roots of the ABC Model

THE HUMAN ENVIRONMENT AS A FORCE FIELD

Scientific concepts emerge from inferences associated with empirical events. For example, Newton developed his laws of gravity from observing the "behavior" of falling objects, such as apples. Kurt Lewin, in his topological psychology, theorized that the human environment was analogous to an electromagnetic field with positive and negative forces to which adaption, simplistically stated, consisted of adient (approach) behavior to positively valent aspects and abient (avoidance) behavior to negatively valent situations[68]. Schematically represented by vectors having both directional and magnitudinal components, these goal-directed behaviors in Figure 2.1 symbolically become the environmental referents for the terms motive, emotion, conflict, and stress as used in this book.

The overall objective of Lewin's topological and vector psychology was to apply mathematical principles stated in vector and topological language to the problem of explaining personality and adjustment. This book, however, is written at a different conceptual level[69]. Although Lewinian terms are used frequently throughout, in the interest of pragmatism, they are not defined mathematically, but instead are defined operationally in terms of environmental referents. Accordingly, some definitions of selected concepts pertaining to Figure 2.1 follow: At the outset, the schematic symbolizes the interaction of a person's perceptual or phenomenal field as well as his/her physical field, the former defined in the Lewinian sense as the totality of objects or events which are directly experienced at any one moment, and the latter as the universe consisting of units of matter (electrons, atoms, molecules, and so on)[70].

The perceptions or meanings associated with stimuli, an integral part of the phenomenal field insofar as the ABC model is concerned, are derived from the sensory data associated with the physical field at a given time. These perceptions,

Figure 2.1
Human Phenomenal Environment Depicted as a Force Field

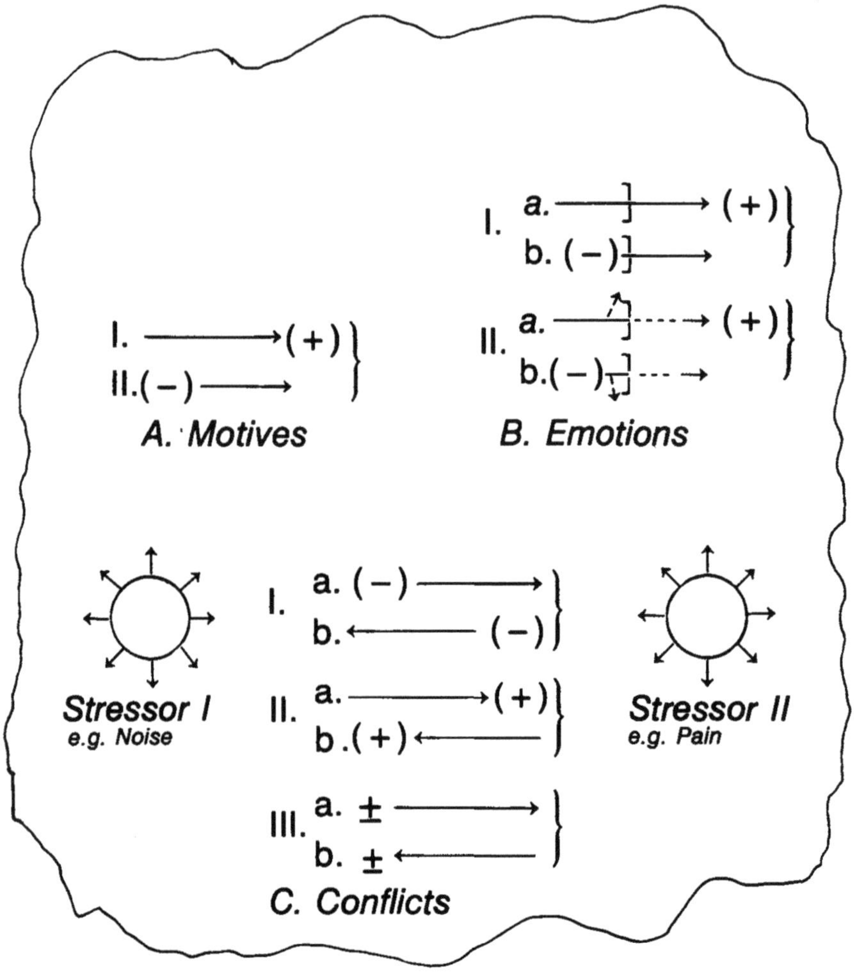

Goal-directed behavior (motives) are symbolized by vectors. A. Motives: I (+), positively valent motive, II (−), negatively valent motive. B. Emotions: Ia and Ib positive emotions, IIa and IIb negative emotions. C. Conflicts: Ia and Ib double avoidance, IIa and IIb double approach, and IIIa and IIIb double approach/avoidance.

in turn, take on valence or value-related properties, positive or negative, when associated with the attainment or non-attainment of appropriate goals or outcomes.

Motives are represented by vectors in Figure 2.1. These vectors represent the direction and magnitude of goal-directed behavior within the force field. The properties of motives are inferred from the interrelationship between the NPP (Need Prepotency Profile) and the valence characteristics of the correlated goals or satisfiers present in the field at a given time (AI and AII). Although intrinsically related to motives, emotions, on the other hand, refer to the organismic response patterns resulting from the backlash effects of environmental impediments or barriers upon the adapting person. Positive (+) emotions (elation, pleasurable excitement) tend to occur in environmental circumstances in which barriers to ongoing behavior are perceived as nonexistent, permeable, or circumventable. Stated in the language of physics, positive emotions occur in environmental conditions in which the inertia of the barrier or impediment is minimal and the momentum of the motivational vector is sustained (BIa and BIb in Figure 2.1). In contrast, negative emotions (anxiety, fear, panic, embarrassment, and so on) occur in environmental situations in which the barriers are, or at least are perceived as being, impermeable, semipermeable, or noncircumventable. That is, motivational momentum is minimal and environmental inertia is maximal (BIIa and BIIb).

It is both interesting and informative that the basis for labeling emotions as positive (+) or negative (−) stems from the findings of K. M. B. Bridges [19] in regard to the emergence of emotions in neonates. The common observation that persons generally (not always) tend to seek environmental situations that evoke positive emotions (humor, joy) and, conversely, tend to avoid circumstances that produce negative emotions (fear, anger) further supports this point of view.

Also noteworthy in this context is the fact that emotional reactivity, the most important component of POSR, is *passive*; that is, the perceptions or meanings associated with environmental cues cause the emotions for the person. Stated simply, emotions, both positive and negative, result from the *back-action* of the environment upon the person[87]. Unlike a person's voluntarily lifting a hand or speaking, under ordinary circumstances, the same person cannot become fearful, elated, or embarrassed at will. There may be a few exceptions, for example, some professional actors and actresses, cast in highly emotional roles, such as are found in Shakespearian plays, for example, may with the help of stage make-up turn on overt signs of anger, fear, or joy at will. However, it is doubtful that the subjective or affective component of these emotions are truly present at that time.

A related aspect of emotional processes that is unique in behavioral science is the fact that emotions, like the perception of color, are qualitative dimensions of experience, not the total experience. For example, define the color red or green. The illumination engineer defines these colors in terms of frequency and wavelength of the color stimulus. The color stimulus, however, can more completely be described by pointing to a red sweater or to green grass. Also, the abstraction "love" as a positive emotion has little meaning. But, if an object or a delineative phrase is added to "love," love for a person, a musical composition, or a painting, for instance, the emotional experience of "love" becomes much more descriptive. Similarly, what is fear or anger or POSR for that matter? None of these emotions can be completely defined without pointing to a "feared" or anger-provoking situation or object. Too, POSR cannot be completely described without referencing the environmental situation (person, place, or thing) that evoked the stress reactivity in the first place. These environmental situations—persons, places, or things—that cause POSR of differing levels of intensity, are called *stressors* in this book.

So what are the implications of this theoretical diversion into the psychology of emotions for this text on stress? As the cartoon character Pogo has said, "We have found the enemy and it is us"; we have found the blind spot in many past studies of stress, namely, focusing too much on stress reactions and too little on those aspects of the environment that cause stress, the stressors. In anticipation, Chapter 9 of this text contains a detailed discussion of SIRO (Stressor Identification and Rank Ordering), a new procedure for the identification and evaluation of the stressors present in a given environmental situation at a given time.

The term "conflict" as depicted in Figure 2.1 refers to motivational vectors channelized in opposite directions (CIa, CIb, CIIa, CIIb, CIIIa, and CIIIb). Frequently, intense motives in opposition resulting in a conflict situation are reacted to as impermeable barriers (stressors), the result being the emergence of negative emotions or POSR in most cases. The often-heard expressions "between a rock and a hard place" and "between the devil and the deep blue sea" would seem to apply to one of the three types of conflicts (Fig. 2.1), the double avoidance conflict (CIa and CIb). Equally stress-evoking perhaps are the other two types of conflicts, double approach (CIIa and CIIb) and double approach/avoidance (CIIIa and CIIIb) conflicts.

Finally, defined as a cluster of forces within a force field, the two kinds of stressors are represented in Figure 2.1 as explosive mines, symbolically indicating their fulminating potential. Noteworthy is the fact that the direction of the vectors emanating from the two categories of stressors, presented in Figure 2.1 are abient, suggesting that, in general, stressors tend to evoke negative emotions and, consequently, avoidance motivation.

Theories or models in science are explanatory frames of reference that, to be useful, must be empirically proven to shed some light on important facts associated with the phenomena of interest, in this instance, stress. Theories are developed to answer the question *why*. In the area of stress, why are some stress-related variables highly intercorrelated, some positively and some negatively, whereas other variables are uncorrelated? Why do these and other variables tend to show significant interperson variation as well as intraperson variation over time? Why and by what mechanisms do certain psychophysiological processes tend to predict individual differences in stress reactivity, whereas others have no predictive validity?

In this context, the ABC model of *stress* to be discussed in the following chapter is directed toward five major objectives: (1) to show that the major components of *stress* or POSR are similar to negative emotions, which, in turn, result from the opposition of two forces, goal-directed behavior and the inertia or resistance to this channelized energy caused by environmental impediments or barriers (stressors); (2) to suggest an approach for identifying and rank ordering environmental stressors in terms of their SEP; (3) to suggest simple, self-administratable procedures for preventing excessive POSR build up; (4) to develop techniques for the assessment of individual differences in SCC; and (5) to identify effective preventive and therapeutic techniques, in some cases of the "do-it-yourself" variety, for reducing and sustaining an adaptable level of POSR once it has approached debilitating and possibly pathological intensity.

3

The ABC Model of Stress

A model is a representation of the interrelationship of objects, processes, or events. For example, a topographical map graphically represents the physical configuration of a terrestrial region. To be useful, or at least heuristic, a model of *stress* should not only indicate the interrelationships of crucial variables, but also must at least imply the direction of causality culminating in *stress*, or POSR, the term of choice in this book[56].

Figure 3.1 might more appropriately be labeled "The ABC Model of Stress and *Motivation*" since, according to the model, stress is unlikely to occur for an unmotivated person, one who is dead or deeply anesthetized, to cite some extreme examples. The stage is set for acute or chronic stress, or POSR in this model, when the goal-directed behavior of a person (B_I or B_{II}) loses momentum as a result of encounters with environmental barriers or impediments to achieving highly valent goals, reinforcers, or consequences ("C" in the model). To the degree that these motivational vectors, either positive or negative, are blocked or impeded by the environmental barriers or stressors, to that degree will negative emotional reactions (such as anxiety, fear, panic, or depression, i.e., POSR) occur. Stated differently, the ABC model implies that the term stress (POSR) has as its referent complex emotional patterns, made up of at least six classes of processes resulting from the opposition of two forces, one a goal-directed contingency, and the other an immediate or anticipated environmental barrier to this ongoing activity. In short, stress or POSR consists of the reaction pattern resulting from "an irresistible (more or less) force meeting an immovable (more or less) object." Considering Figures 2.1 and 3.1 together, numerous practical examples of this paradigm are rather obvious: for instance, the repeated failure of a well-motivated undergraduate to be accepted in a doctoral program, or the death of a loved one, or repeated occupational failure (BIIa in Figure 2.1).

Figure 3.1
ABC Model of Stress

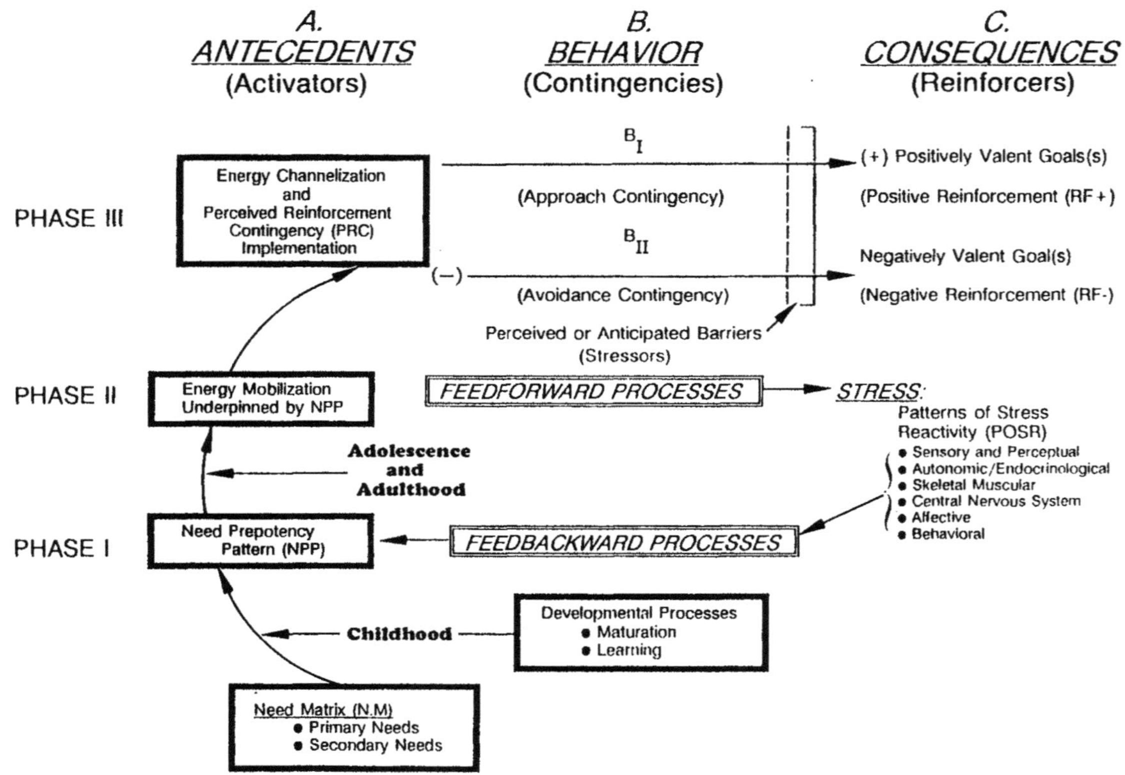

Additional examples of a rise in the intensity of POSR resulting from blocked avoidance contingencies (BIIb in Figure 2.1) might be a person's experiencing intense, intractable pain from a chronic disease or injury, or the inability to avoid paying an IRS debt far exceeding one's available resources. In some cases, a common avoidance contingency for the resultant POSR, particularly the affective component, is the consumption of sedative or mood-altering drugs, including alcohol. Too, chronic anxiety, depression, and phobias are common components of the POSR resulting from blocked or impeded avoidance as well as approach behavior.

In graduate-level stress seminars for the past eleven years, the author has used what has come to be called the RBD (rubber band demonstration) to define the concept of stress as depicted by the ABC model. Briefly, the RBD consists of first asking the members of the seminar for a show of hands of those who would like to receive a grade "A" in the course. As expected, unanimity reigns; all hands are raised with enthusiasm, as it is a generally accepted fact among graduate students that a high grade point average is a *sine qua non* for being accepted in most doctoral programs, as well as for being hired by many prospective employers.

The second step in the RBD is to give each student a regular office-type rubber band. The bands vary greatly in thickness, length, and elasticity. Next, the students are asked to stretch the band over the *back* of his/her preferred hand, twist it *once*, and loop one end around the thumb and the other end around the little finger. Then, the instructions are given as follows: "Your task is to remove the band *without* using your nonpreferred hand or without rubbing the 'bound' hand across your body or anything else. The time limit is five minutes." At this point, in an improvised manner, the positive valence (*see* Glossary) of the goal (to remove the band according to the rules) is established by clearly stating that the person or persons who authentically remove the band within the five-minute time limit will be guaranteed a course grade of "A." "So, go ahead, you have five minutes by my stopwatch to get the band off your hand. Ready, START!"

During the next five minutes, there is characteristically a great deal of noise, grunts, sighing, and some cursing; the preferred hand is twisted, contorted, fingers clawing, wrist flexed up and down, and so on. A great deal of chatter goes on, some laughing, some angry comments—all in all, much confusion but only *one* student out of more than 250 seminar registrants has ever gotten the band off within the constraints imposed.

By analogy, the RBD attempts to simulate the phases in the ABC model describing the processes involved in producing POSR (Figure 3.1). Looking at the model, it is seen that Phase I involves the manner in which a need within the NPP becomes prepotent or compelling. In RBD, as used in the stress seminar, the need for achievement is made prepotent by raising the possibility of earning an "A" in the course. Phase II, the energy mobilization phase, is accomplished in the RBD implemented in the seminar by stating and restating the fact that grade point average is a prime consideration for admission to many doctoral programs and is also looked upon as a very important qualification for being hired by most prospective employers in the world of work. This "sales" strategy serves not only to mobilize energy and enthusiasm, but also as a means to enhance the valence or importance of the goal of the exercise.

Still looking at Figure 3.1 Phase III, the energy channelization and contingency selection and implementation phase, is analogized in RBD by clearly describing the behavioral activity necessary for goal attainment, that is, removal of the band. The spelling out of the reinforcement contingencies *necessary* to reach the positively valent goal completes the "A" or antecedent segment of the ABC sequence.

The "B" or contingency implementation part of ABC is being carried out during the five-minute activity period of the RBD. Quite early into the five-minute time interval, most (all?) of the students typically begin to realize that goal attainment may be impossible, that is, the blockage of the strong goal-directed behavior is being anticipated, and, upon approaching the end of the five-minute period, is fully realized. In the language of the ABC model, there are no available PRC's or ARC's (perceived reinforcement contingencies and anticipated reinforcement contingencies in that order) by means of which the desired outcome could be realized. In other words, the inertia of the barrier (stressor) and the momentum of the high-energy motivational vector in opposition have produced the setting for the POSR to occur. The POSR that is likely to occur will be of varying intensity from one person to another and will involve different patterns of the six classes of reactivity processes making up POSR as listed in Figure 3.1.

Not only do the students participating in the RBD experience the POSR resulting from the stressors being imposed upon a positively valent motivational vector, but also the POSR resulting from blockage of a negatively valent vector as well. This is the purpose of the rubber bands being of different widths, lengths, and elasticity. The bands pinch sharply and actually produce quite intense pain, certainly irritation, during the five-minute time span, the degree of discomfort depending upon the three characteristics of the band itself. This feature of the RBD is meant to demonstrate individual differences in the affective component of the POSR that the same perceived stressor may evoke. Moreover, the degree of impermeability of the stressor or barrier to goal attainment can be increased by requiring more than one twist of the rubber band stretched across the back of the participant's hand. Thus, both the B_I approach contingency and the B_{II} avoidance contingency depicted in Figure 3.1 are, by analogy, simulated in the rubber band demonstration.

The RBD can of course be used to explain the dynamics of stress as depicted in the ABC model in contexts other than a seminar on stress. For example, RBD should be quite effective for this purpose in many stress management seminars directed toward salespeople, parishioners, or housewives—almost anyone. The only change in the RBD procedure necessary would be the incentive(s) by which high positive valence is attached to the goal or outcome. For instance, job promotion, significant monetary reward, time off, or a bundle of lottery tickets should be quite sufficient for that purpose.

Now for a more technical discussion of the ABC model of stress. Implicit in the RBD is the assumption that the dynamics of POSR depicted in the ABC model are intrinsically associated with the cyclic nature of motivation. The infant is born with a number of *needs* (deficiencies) that, at the outset at least, are mainly primary needs; that is, their satisfaction is vital for survival. Examples of these primary or basic needs are: need for oxygen, food, fluid, waste elimination, and sleep. The prepotency of these needs is also cyclic, for example, fifteen to twenty-five breaths per minute or, as parents of their firstborn neonate can aptly attest, the sleep/wakefulness cycle, the hungry/satiated, and the dry/wet phases of the new arrival[51].

The development of appropriate contingencies for satisfying some of these primary needs and almost all of the secondary needs in later childhood involves both maturation and learning processes. Throughout childhood into adulthood, additional needs, mainly secondary, develop. For the most part, contingencies for these needs are learned. Examples of these secondary needs are: need for affiliation, self-esteem, achievement, and later on, status and power.

Two major motivational theorists, A. H. Maslow and C. P. Alderfer, assume that the prepotent needs in the NPP at a given time are a function of those needs that are or are not satisfied at that time[1, 77]. Along similar lines, the basic assumption underpinning Phase I of the ABC model is that the NPP fluctuates from time to time, varying with (a) the maturational level of the person, (b) the satiation state of the needs functioning at a given time, (c) the environmental antecedents or activators present ("A" in Figure 3.1), and (d) in particular, the nature of the prevailing stressors existing at that time[3, 88].

Phase II, the energy mobilization, arousal, or drive phase of the motivation cycle, results from "need tension," to borrow a Lewinian term. It results from the synergistic effect of the NPP and causes the person to seek out environmental antecedents or activators with which cues for action have been associated through learning processes. These learned acts are called PRC's, having a significant probability of resulting in the achievement of high valent goals or the consummation of satisfiers appropriate for the prevailing NPP.

This leads to Phase III, the contingency(ies) selection and implementation phase, resulting in goal-directed behavior represented by the (+) and (−) vectors in Figure 3.1 (B_I and B_{II}). A fictitious example of the five-step sequence (NPP-energized, → energy-mobilization, → contingency-selection, → contingency-implementation, → goal-attainment) for a typical person in the work place might be as follows: a mechanical engineer, noting that his/her income is insufficient, at the same time, discovers that a managing engineering position carrying a significant salary increase will be vacant two years hence (the "A" in ABC). Subsequently, an NPP with, for example, NAch (Need for Achievement) as the highest in prepotency, becomes dominant[78]. Phase I then leads directly to Phase II, resulting in energy being mobilized to identify the local institutions featuring eve-

Figure 3.2
Consequences "C" in ABC Model

Affective Context (AC)	Consequences (C)	
	C-Imposed	C-Withheld
Positive (+AC)	CI_1 Positive Reinforcement (RF+)	CW_1 Positive Punishment (Pu+)
Negative (-AC)	CI_2 Negative Punishment (Pu-)	CW_2 Negative Reinforcement (RF-)

ning graduate programs pursuant to an MBA degree, a stated requirement for the job. Phase III follows during which PRC's and ARC's are evaluated, the result being the selection of a sequence of contingencies that support high expectancies to lead to degree attainment. For example, the "B" sequence in ABC might include long-term activities, such as arduous study schedules, class attendance, test taking, and so on. With diploma in hand, the engineer then applies and is interviewed for the position. If our legendary engineer gets the job, one would predict that positive emotions (elation, pleasurable excitement) would occur, since relatively impermeable barriers have been removed, overcome, or circumvented (BIa, Figure 2.1). Conversely, should he/she be rejected for the position, the barriers to these goal-directed contingencies would be buttressed or new ones erected (BIIa, Figure 2.1). POSR of varying degrees of intensity would quite likely occur as the result of this blockage.

There are four broad categories of consequences or outcomes, "C" in ABC, that may result from our fictitious engineer's carrying out the long-term series of contingencies terminating in his being considered for the position. These are presented in a 2 × 2 matrix format in Figure 3.2.

It should be acknowledged at the outset that this classification of behavioral consequences and their contingent behavior is obliquely related to one of the oldest principles of American psychology, namely, E. L. Thorndike's Law of Effect[117]. Simply stated, this principle holds that the association between stimulus and response (A and B in the ABC model) is influenced by the effects or consequences of what a person does: if the outcome is associated with pleasure (+AC), "satisfiers" for Thorndike, the behavior tends to be repeated, whereas, if it is associated with unpleasant consequences (−AC), "punishers," the behavior tends to drop out. Accordingly, the contingency(ies) producing the consequences in cells CI_1, positive reinforcement, RF+, tends to be repeated. Diagonally opposite CI_1 is CW_2, negative reinforcement or RF−. Similar to an approach contingency, an avoidance contingency that results in unpleasant consequences (−AC) being withheld tends also to be repeated.

There are, however, two additional possible consequences: CW_1 and CI_2, positive and negative punishment, Pu+ and Pu−, respectively. Simply stated, Pu+, sometimes called delayed RF (reinforcement), is a planned reinforcement schedule whereby RF+ is withheld until the desired contingency occurs. Repetition of this contingent behavior is likely in this situation. Contrarily, Pu−, diagonally opposite CW_1 (Pu+) in the matrix schematic, involves the imposition of conditions causing −AC as a consequence of the completion of a specific contingency. Immediate suppression of this reinforcement contingency usually occurs but is likely to reappear later[112].

To continue the fictitious example of the promotion-seeking engineer, the upper left cell, CI_1, positive reinforcement (RF+) describes the situation in which the employer hired the engineer. As a result of the +AC associated with this outcome, the new incumbent in the position under discussion will have learned that his/her selection of contingencies had been essentially correct. On the other hand, let us suppose that the prospective employer declared the applicant ineligible for the position, the outcome in the lower left cell, CI_2(Pu−). This outcome would describe an event that would tend to invalidate past contingency selection. Moreover, the occurrence of Pu−, the CI_2 outcome, not only suggests that the contingencies leading to CI_2(Pu−) were inappropriate, but also would likely result in the precipitation of intense POSR. In addition, POSR would also tend to be sustained for the job seeker by the effect of Pu+ (CW_1), consisting of withholding RF+ until the engineer carried out a set of contingencies that would result in his/her meeting the qualification standards for the job.

Finally, negative reinforcement (RF−), cell CW_2, consisting of contingency reinforcement by means of *avoidance* of −AC, might conceivably occur in a situation in which our engineer, upon learning that his/her present company's planned reorganization would result in his/her being involuntarily terminated in his/her present job and the new position being eliminated at the same time, abruptly adopts the contingency of resigning in order to *avoid* the chagrin and the concomitant POSR of being fired.

The dynamics of avoidance motivation (RF−) are extremely important for the study of stress, so much so that additional examples of the phenomenon are indicated at this point. At the level of laboratory science, for example, there is substantial evidence that avoidance motivation is very strong and is sustained for long periods of time. One early experiment involved the conditioning of dogs to avoid mild electrical shock when a buzzer sounded ten seconds before the onset of shock. The avoidance response consisted of jumping a hurdle to reach a nonshock compartment. This jumping contingency, reinforced by RF−, was learned in a very few trials. Moreover, the association between the buzzer signaling "shock is coming" and the hurdle-jumping behavior persisted for months, even for some of the animals that had undergone surgical removal of the ganglionic chain of the sympathetic nervous system, part of the nervous system related to fear reactivity[113].

More mundane examples of the function of avoidance or RF− motivation for human adjustment are plentiful: The set of contingencies required to complete and file the proper IRS forms on April 15 is, for many citizens, motivated to *avoid* paying a penalty, the motivation to stop at a red stoplight even with clear intersections is quite likely motivated to *avoid* being arrested, or a more poignant example might be the billions of dollars spent annually on tranquilizers, analgesics, and other pain-killing medication, including alcohol and other recreational drugs—all used to *avoid* pain, anxiety, and other affective components of POSR.

Feedback results from the AC (affective context) associated with the consequences of goal-directed behavior. As indicated in Figure 3.1, feedback effects generally result in modification of the NPP. For example, the positive feedback from our engineer's being hired for the highly desired position (RF+) might result in her/his joining the country club to satisfy affiliative needs, heretofore low on the NPP. On the other hand, being rejected for the job (Pu−) might have negative feedback effects on the prevailing NPP; for example, engineering management may have lost its positive valence for him or her. As a result, opening a machine tooling shop might become a contingency for some ego-supportive needs that have suddenly assumed enhanced prepotency in the NPP. In summary, positive feedback tends to be associated with +AC, and contingencies resulting in RF+ or RF−. Conversely, negative feedback tends to be associated with −AC, and contingencies associated with Pu+ and Pu− outcomes.

There are several categories of positive reinforcement (RF+): material RF (salary, profit sharing, retirement plans), social RF, such as enhanced status and prestige, and +AC itself as, for example, when one experiences a sense of accomplishment in passing a test, hitting a home run, winning the lottery, and so on. Still another class of RF+, particularly appropriate for children, is called activity RF, or "grandmother's rule," an example of which might be the advice given to the little leaguer, "first you mow the lawn, then you can play baseball." Grandmother's rule has been expanded over the years as the so-called Premack Principle. Simply stated, this principle is "an activity ranked low on the preference hierarchy may be effectively reinforced by an activity ranked higher on the same scale." A simple example of this principle might be the admonition to the reluctant sixth grader who conforms to the modern stereotype of the "tube junkie," "*only* after you have completed your homework will you be allowed to watch TV." In this case, the Premack Principle is concerned with the consequence "C" in Figure 3.1 applied as positive punishment (Pu+), consisting of withholding RF+, the highly desirable contingency of TV viewing, until, and only until, the less desirable contingency of completing the homework assignment materializes.

CLASSES OF PROCESSES MAKING UP POSR (PATTERNS OF STRESS REACTIVITY)

To reiterate, in the development of the ABC model, it was assumed that the term *stress* refers to emotional reactivity patterns, negative emotions for the most part, resulting from immediately perceived or anticipated environmental barriers to goal-directed behavior. These barriers or impediments are called stressors. The term POSR (Patterns of Stress Reactivity) has been coined to refer to the reactivity patterns caused by these stressors.

Since the major components of POSR are emotional in nature, in order to comprehend the dynamics of POSR, it is essential to understand the emotional processes themselves. Consequently, a brief diversion into the psychophysiology of emotions follows[128].

THE PSYCHOPHYSIOLOGY OF EMOTIONS

Emotions are a class of organismic processes resulting from the interaction of environmental resistances (or lack of resistance) to goal-directed behavior[87]. Emotions result from the momentum of goal-directed activity counteracting with the inertial characteristics of environmental impediments or barriers. If the environmental resistance decreases or is removed, positive emotions, such as joy, pleasurable excitement, and so forth, occur. On the other hand, if resistance remains steady or increases, negative emotions (fear, anger, embarrassment) tend to occur. As stated earlier, the labeling of emotions as positive or negative stems from the tendency in most instances for a person to seek out and approach aspects of the environment that tend to evoke positive (+) emotions and to avoid circumstances that result in negative (−) emotions. Mentioned in Chapter 2, but worthy of repeating here, is the fact that emotions are the *passive* or backlash effects of the environment, that is, they are reactive, not active responses to environmental situations. Except for a few professional thespians, a person has the ability to scream or kick the wall voluntarily, but cannot, at will, be "happy," "sad," or "angry." Instead, it is the meanings derived from perceptual patterns associated with environmental objects or situations that *cause* emotional reactivity, including POSR.

Positive and negative attitudes toward various aspects of the environment, including people, are also developed by essentially the same dynamism, but there are exceptions to this simplistic explanation of the polarity of emotions and attitudes. For example, such people as Evel Knieval deliberately sought out fear-inducing situations, for example, jumping the Grand Canyon on a rocket-assisted motorcycle. Presumably, the superimposed positively valent reinforcer (millions of dollars) tended to support the jumping contingency and suppress somewhat the fear involved.

Thus, knowledge of the perceptual properties of the environment becomes essential for understanding emotions. It follows that the mechanisms by which a person's cognitive frame of reference develops are intrinsically related to the sensory and perceptual processes themselves. In turn, sensory and perceptual processes are inherently related to the structural and functional characteristics of selected regions of the nervous system. Therefore, in order to round out the

Figure 3.3
The Human Nervous System

1. Central Nervous System

    1.1 Brain

        1.11 Cerebral Cortex--3 Functional Areas: sensory, motor, and association areas.

        1.12 Cerebellum, Brain Steam

    1.2 Spinal Cord

2. Peripheral Nervous System

    2.1 Autonomic Nervous System (ANS)--a motor system: it controls the internal environment.

        2.11 Sympathetic Nervous System (SNS)

        2.12 Parasympathetic nervous System (PNS)

    2.2 Somatic Nervous System--processes involved in the interaction between the internal and external environment.

    2.21 Motor System

    2.22 Sensory System

        2.221 Exteroceptive Senses (External or peripheral senses) vision, audition, and chemical senses: gustation and olfaction. Skin or somaesthetic senses: tactual, pain, and the thermal senses of cold and warmth.

        2.222 Interoceptive Senses (Internal or deep senses) Proprioceptive Senses: Kinesthetic (joints and muscular movement) and vestibular senses (equilibrium). Visceral or Organ Senses: endoderm organs such as the gastro-intestinal tract and kidneys.

study of emotions, a brief decimally coded outline of the human nervous system is shown in Figure 3.3.

The expression, almost a truism, "no perception without sensation" accents the relevance of both the exteroceptive and interoceptive senses (2.221 and 2.222 in the outline above) for understanding the development of the percepts or meanings associated with environmental objects or situations. These patterns of sensory inputs, called sensations, in turn, are transmitted at speeds up to 100 meters (300 feet) per second by the neural tracts in the spinal cord to the brain. There, by means of complex neuronal processes in the sensory and association areas of the cerebral cortex, perceptions are formed to become the sensorium, a principal component of a waking person's consciousness at a given time.

Besides sensations resulting from the stimuli impinging on the receptors for the ten sensory modalities listed in the outline (coded 2.22), there are several other factors affecting perception in a given instance: attention or expectancy, prevailing NPP, and the learning residue of past experience, to name a few. To capsulize the discussion of perception as it relates to stress, the sum total of these interacting perceptions becomes the building blocks for the cognitive frame of reference underpinning the interpretation of a given set of stressors, which, in turn, causes the emotional reactive patterns we have labeled POSR.

Perhaps the most important nervous system components of emotions are the response patterns associated with the ANS (autonomic nervous system), coded 2.1 in the outline above[4]. As the word "autonomic" connotes, this motor system is largely involuntary as contrasted with the SMS (somatic motor system), which, in the waking state at least, is more or less under voluntary control (2.2). However, it may be well to point out that recent findings in the area of biofeedback technology clearly demonstrate that by means of behavioral modification techniques many ANS functions (e.g., heart rate and blood pressure) can, to an extent, be brought under voluntary control.

The ANS exerts motor control on the person's internal environment and involves smooth muscle responses, whereas the SMS involves the interaction between the external and internal environments and involves only striated muscle responses. The ANS is composed of two somewhat antagonistic subsystems whose anatomical and functional characteristics are compared in Table 3.1[128].

In general, most organs are enervated by both PNS (parasympathetic nervous system) and SNS (sympathetic nervous system) nerve fibers. Exceptions occur, however; for example, the nonheat regulatory sweat glands in the palms of the hand are enervated by sympathetic cholinergic (vice adrenergic) fibers only. As a result, these sweat glands do not react to adrenalin injection as do most of the SNS-enervated organs. Similarly, pilomotor response (goose pimples) results only from SNS/cholinergic activity.

As is seen in (d) in Table 3.1, most SNS postganglionic fibers are adrenergic, that is, they produce adrenalin-like substances at the synapses. By comparison, *all* preganglionic fibers in both the SNS and PNS as well as *all* postganglionic fibers of the PNS are cholinergic (i.e., produce acetylcholine at the synapses).

These anomalous relationships between the two branches of the ANS and the substances found at their synapses and along their ganglionic fibers have some important functional implications for the study of the emotional component of stress. Accordingly, comparison "j" in Table 3.1, the relative dissipation rates of adrenalin from the SNS and acetylcholine from the PNS, is noteworthy from the standpoint of the differences in the duration of negative as compared to

Table 3.1
Comparison of the Anatomical and Functional Characteristics of the Two Subsystems of the Autonomic Nervous System

SUB-SYSTEM I: SYMPATHETIC	SUB SYSTEM II: PARASYMPATHETIC
ANATOMICAL	
a. Thoraco-lumbar	a. Cranio-sacral
b. Synapses in the sympathetic chain; preganglionic nerves are short with ganglia along the spinal cord	b. Preganglionic nerves long, originating in brain stem (cranial nerves III –mesencephalon (mid-brain), VII, IX --medulla and X, and in sacral motor roots, ganglia are near enervated organs
FUNCTIONAL	
a. Sympathetic Nervous System (SNS), "in sympathy with"	a. Parasympathetic Nervous System (PNS) "around SNS", above and below spinal cord
b. Sympathetico-adrenal	b. Vago-insulin
c. Adrenergic, react to adrenalin	c. Cholinergic, react to acetylcholine
d. Postganglionic fibers liberate substance similar to epinephrine (produced by the adrenal medulla) and called Sympathin, Sympathin I (inhibitory), Sympathin II (excitatory)	d. Postganglionic fibers liberate acetylcholine
e. Diffuse, generalized response	e. Specific, particularized response
f. Catabolic (inhomeostatic), disequilibrating	f. Anabolic (homeostatic) vegetative, equilibrating
g. Constitutes a positive feedback loop, i.e., input positively correlated with output, a runaway (berserk) system	g. Constitutes a negative feedback loop, i.e., input negatively correlated with output, a stabilizing system
h. Associated with negative emotions	h. Associated with positive emotions
i. Analogous to an auto distributor "short out"	i. Distributor fires in sequence
j. Adrenaline-like substances dissipate very slowly	j. Acetylcholine dissipates rapidly

See glossary for definition of terms.

positive emotional reactions. These differences in dissipation rates of adrenalin and acetylcholine may in part account for the well-known fact that hours, even days, after an intense fear-inducing experience has occurred, a near-miss traffic accident, for example, symptoms of SNS reactivity, such as heart palpitation, palmar sweating, and pallor, still persist. In contrast, the concomitants of a PNS reaction associated with the euphoria of an event, such as winning the lottery or passing Ph.D. orals, quickly subside minutes after the event has occurred. The generalized, diffuse nature of the SNS reaction compared to the specific, particularized PNS response (''e'' in Table 3.1) provides additional support for the same proposition. Finally, comparative statements ''h'' in Table 3.1 associate SNS reactivity with negative emotions and PNS overflow with positive emotions.

As has been discussed earlier, most of the major components of POSR are similar to those found in negative emotions. Thus, knowledge of SNS function in particular takes on singular importance for the study of stress.

Another difference between negative, adrenergic emotional reactivity (fear, −AC) and positive, cholinergic emotional reactivity (joy, +AC) is the difference in the Pavlovian conditionability of the two kinds of emotions. For instance, the experience of returning years later to the intersection where you witnessed a loved one's being killed in a terrible car accident still induces some degree of the past anguish. But, returning months later to the stage of the amphitheater where, after years of study and personal sacrifice, you had experienced elation and a sense of achievement upon receiving your doctoral hood, results in little or no emotional response of any kind. Similarly, why does a return visit to the chapel wherein you were happily married six months earlier fail to evoke any of the positive emotions previously experienced? On the other hand, returning to the same chapel wherein you had attended the funeral of your young child years before causes the arousal of some degree of the past distress. In short, it appears that the classical conditioning of negative emotional reactivity to the environmental situation that produced it occurs much more readily than does the conditioning of positive emotions to the associated emotion-inducing circumstance. It may be that this observation accounts in part for the persistence of the residue of intense stress reactions since negative emotions are a major component of the associated POSR.

Although mostly covert, ANS reactivity patterns in some instances have some overt peripheral components as well. Table 3.2 demonstrates the antagonistic characteristics of both overt and covert SNS and PNS reactivity as related to selected organs and body structures. Again, this comparison is indexed in decimals.

At the outset, it should be noted in Table 3.2 that some of these peripheral indices of stress reactivity are directly observable, for example, during a post-stress interview. For instance, with the illumination level constant, the pupillary response of the eye (1.1 in Table 3.2) usually dilates in a stress situation and contracts in a nonstress situation[132]. Also, because of the vasoconstrictive and vasodilatory functions of the ANS, skin tends to become pale and cold during SNS stimulation, but becomes flushed and warm with PNS stimulation (or the absence of SNS overflow).

Many of the remaining antagonistic indicators of SNS and PNS reactivity, although not directly observable, are readily measurable, for example, heart rate, blood pressure, skin conductivity, skin temperature, and so on (codes 3, 4, and 11 in Table 3.2). Still other indices, such as urinary epinephrine and other hormonal levels, blood sugar concentration, and the expiratory and inspiratory volume of the lungs can also be measured by laboratory techniques.

One final medical point should be made regarding the SNS and PNS comparisons in Table 3.2. The mechanisms by which disease-related conditions may be exacerbated by acute or chronic POSR are suggested by the functional com-

Table 3.2
Functional Relationships of SNS and PNS Activity to Selected Organs and Body Structures

Structure or Organ	SNS	PNS
1. Eye		
1.1 Iris	Dilation of pupil	Contraction
1.2 Ciliary Muscle	Relaxation of ciliary muscles accommodation for distance vision	Contraction of ciliary muscles for close viewing
2. Bronchial Tubes	Dilation	Constriction
3. Heart	Heart rate acceleration; Blood pressure increase	Heart rate decreases Blood pressure drops
4. Blood Vessels		
4.1 Cerebral	Constriction	Dilation
4.2 Coronary Arteries	Dilation	Constriction
4.3 Abdominal and Pelvic Viscera	Constriction	Varies
4.4 External Genitalia	Constriction of blood vessels	Dilation of blood vessels
5. Stomach		
5.1 Muscles	Depresses activity	Increase activity
5.2 Glands	Decreases secretion	Increase secretion
6. Liver	Increases glycogenolysis	Increases glycogenesis
7. Visceral Muscle of Intestine	Depresses peristalsis Relaxes sphincters	Increases peristalsis Contracts sphincters
8. Adrenal Medulla	Secretion of epinephrine (Adrenalin)	Non-reactive
9. Sweat Glands (heat regulatory)	Secretion	Varies
10. Sweat Glands (non-heat regulatory); palms of hands, upper lip	Secretion	Not enervated by PNS
11. Skin	Cools; pallor occurs Increases Electro-dermal conductance	Warms; redness occurs Non-reactive

parisons of SNS and PNS in Table 3.2. For example, since the SNS component of POSR stimulates glycogenolysis (coded 6 in Table 3.2), stored sugar (glycogen) in the liver is broken down into blood-soluble dextrose, which, in turn, results in elevated blood sugar. Thus, when excreted by the kidneys, sugar shows up in the urine, the common diagnostic sign of diabetes. For the diabetic, therefore, intense POSR may result in the critical requirement for higher dosages of insulin. In short, POSR may disrupt the delicate metabolic balance between sugar and insulin. In extreme cases, insulin insufficiency may cause a diabetic coma. Death could be the end result.

A somewhat paradoxical example of possible untoward medical consequences resulting from intense POSR is the case of the severe asthmatic. SNS reactivity, a major component of POSR, causes the bronchial tubes to dilate (code 2 in Table 3.2), whereas PNS stimulation causes the airways to constrict, which, if extreme, may precipitate the possibly lethal "asthmatic attack." It is interesting, and, as stated above, paradoxical, that the standard treatment for such an attack is to administer an epinephrine-like drug to stimulate the SNS so as to dilate the bronchial tubes and allow adequate oxygen to reach the lungs. In other words, producing an SNS reaction (a stress reaction?) is the standard treatment for a disease process in this case.

One final example of the important relationships between the ANS components of POSR and disease processes is to be found in certain types of male impotency. It is a well-documented fact that the negative emotions fear and anxiety, major components of POSR, are closely related to SNS reactivity (code 4.4 in Table 3.2). As a consequence, because of vasoconstriction, the blood supply to the penis becomes restricted. Thus, the likelihood of penile tumescence and a satisfactory erection is reduced by intense POSR[28].

To reiterate, the purpose of this rather superficial overview of the topic of emotions was to emphasize the central role emotional processes, particularly negative emotions, play in the complex reactivity patterns we have labeled POSR. Although some overlapping of the above discussion is inevitable, the comparison data in Table 3.3 following are an attempt to integrate the major categories of processes constituting the total POSR.

At the outset, it should be emphasized that the various classes of processes contained in Table 3.3 do not always function independently. Quite to the contrary, they interact in complex patterns. For example, both Walter Cannon and later Hans Selye, as part of his General Adaptation Syndrome, demonstrated the hypothalamic-hypophyseal-adrenocortical and the adrenomedullary-hypothalamic axes as they interact with the autonomic nervous system in sustaining homeostasis of bodily functions during stress reactions[21, 105].

Another example of process interaction that provides a partial explanation for the tendency for high-intensity POSR to be of long duration, often eventuating into a chronic decompensated state, is presented schematically in Figure 3.4. These interrelationships have been called the psychosomatic/somatopsychic vicious circle.

An example of this vicious circle might be a middle-aged, MBA-type CEO with significant family responsibilities forced to take early retirement. After a time, with no re-employment possibilities in sight, POSR indicators, such as elevated pulse and blood pressure, tension, insomnia, gastritis, trembling, financial insufficiencies, family turbulence, and depression, begin to appear. The causal direction of this phase of the circle is psycho>soma (psychosomatic),

Table 3.3
Components of POSR (Patterns of Stress Reactivity)

PROCESSES	CHARACTERISTICS		MEASUREMENT STRATEGIES
	Structural	Functional	
A. Cognitive			
1. Sensation	Intero- and Exteroceptive receptors.	Physical stimuli transferred to sensory data.	Bioelectronic measures of stimuli --> receptor interface.
2. Perception	Central Nervous System (CNS) Processes.	Integrates sensory data to yield percepts or meanings.	Subject's response to varying stimulus input.
B. Endocrinological	Glands produce hormones and other substances.	Glandular secretions affect metabolic and neurological processes.	Assay substances in the urine (e.g. catecholamines) and blood (e.g. cholesterol levels).
C. Autonomic Nervous System			
1. Sympathetic	Synapses in Thoraco-Lumbar region. Smooth muscle involved.	Adrenaline system; Inhomeostatic; occurs in negative emotions; occurs in intense POSR (increases blood pressure, pulse, etc.), Distress.	Blood pressure, pulse, skin conductance, pupil diameter, increases measured; drop in skin temperature.
2. Parasympathetic	Preganglionic fibers in cranio-sacral region. Smooth muscle response.	Acetylcholine system; homeostatic; occurs in positive emotions (lowered blood pressure, pulse, etc.), Eustress.	Blood pressure, pulse, skin conductance, pupil diameter, decreases; rise in skin temperature.
D. Skeletal Muscle Response	Involves striated muscle activity (screaming, kicking, running).	Under voluntary control. Locomotion for "fight or flight" reaction.	Direct observation; electromyograms.
E. Affective	CNS and feedback from ANS reactivity.	Unpleasant-Pleasant aspect of emotional reactivity.	Subjective self-report ratings; observer judgements; ANS data.
F. Behavioral	CNS processes involved in decision making and habit formation.	Attitude development; Defense mechanisms and other Stress-coping strategies.	Structured interviews; clinical and psychometric tests; observation.
G. Central Nervous System	Cerebral Cortex, Hypothalamus.	Production of Neurohormones (e.g. serotonin, endorphins, etc.) at the synapses. Electro-physiological changes.	Neurochemical assays of neurohormones; psychometric tests of organicity; electroencephalograms.

Figure 3.4
The Psychosomatic/Somatopsychic Vicious Circle

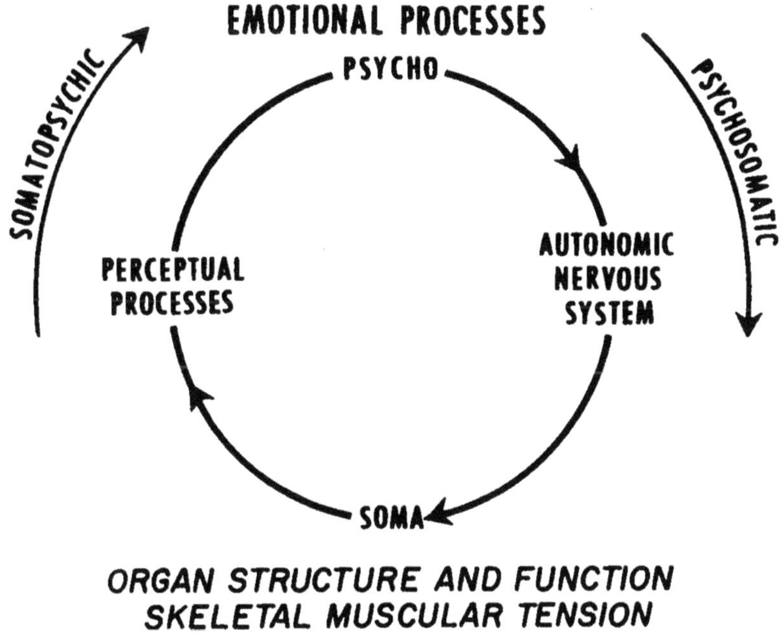

i.e., emotional reactivity is affecting bodily processes via, for the most part, the ANS. In turn, the perceptual awareness of these somatic processes (tightness in the stomach, trembling, palpitating heart) causes the intensity of POSR to increase. The causality in this phase of the circle is in the opposite direction, viz. soma>psycho (somatopsychic). The circle then is back to the first emotional-processes phase progressing to the psychosomatic phase again, and so on. The cycle continues. In computer language, a positive feedback loop, a runaway system, characteristic of negative emotional reactivity generally has eventuated and, as a result, POSR is sustained.

There are at least two different, somewhat overlapping, ways of interrupting or reducing the momentum of the vicious circle. First, by psychopharmacological or psychotherapeutic means, reduce the level of activity in the "Soma" phase of the circle. And/or second, diminish the intensity level of the negative emotional component of the POSR in the "Psycho" phase by providing effective PRC's and ARC's, by means of which the various obstructions or impediments (stressors) to goal-directed activity can be overcome or avoided. These two approaches will be discussed in more detail in Chapter 8, which pertains to the prevention and treatment of stress reactivity.

In a computer age, the somewhat overworked word "system" may be defined as a designed-in linkage of functions coordinated in such a way as to accomplish a specified goal or outcome. Column 3 in Table 3.3, labeled "Functional," describes processes consistent with this definition, in particular if the contents of Table 3.3 are examined in conjunction with the ABC model in Figure 3.1.

Accordingly, a step-by-step verbalization of the dynamics of *stress* or POSR, as developed so far, is possible:

1. As stated earlier, POSR are the results or concomitants of negative emotional reactivity (anxiety, fear, panic, depression).

2. Thus, in Table 3.3 A, B, C–1, D, E, F, and G processes, in different patterns from individual to individual, become the essence of POSR.

3. Perception, the processes by which meanings emanate from patterns of environmental stimuli, is a central concept of Phase III in the ABC model (Figure 3.1), the energy channelization and contingency selection phase. That is, perceptions defining a given stressor or an array of stressors provide the basis for contingency selection. This association between perceived stressors and the contingency possibilities at a given time are called PRC's. Similarly, contingencies that have a high expectancy to be effective for a set of stressors in the future are labeled ARC's. Depending upon an assessment of the degree of permeability of existing environmental barriers or impediments (i.e., stressors), the ABC model allows for the prediction that intense POSR, involving most of the processes described in Table 3.3, have a high probability of occurring when PRC's and ARC's for a given set of stressors are obscure or nonexistent. A simple example would be a turbulent marriage for spouses, both of whom are having extramarital affairs but whose religious convictions prohibit divorce and remarriage. In this situation, meaningful ARC's or PRC's (B in ABC) are seemingly nonexistent. The barriers (stressors) are "seen" as insurmountable. Intense, long-term POSR for both spouses would likely be the end result. Perhaps a more poignant example might be the crew of a submarine lined up single file beneath the escape hatch (A in ABC) of a nuclear submarine incapacitated by a depth charge at 1000 feet seawater depth. In this situation, no realistic PRC's or ARC's would be present, since every crew member would be fully aware that a free ascent from this depth (B in ABC) (thirty atmospheres relative pressure) would most certainty result in air embolism and certain death for every man before, or upon reaching, the surface (C in ABC). In all likelihood, acute POSR would be pervasive within the "sub" crew trapped in this situation[141].

A more common example of these dynamics might be a family man during a financial recession, unemployed, with his monthly payments for the home mortgage, credit card balances, and car loans far exceeding his monthly income. A pile of bills, demanding phone calls from collection agencies, health insurance premiums, and an empty checkbook all become stressors with very high SEP. Insomnia, nervousness, hypertension, stomach and joint pain, and irritability, all symptoms of intense POSR (Table 3.3), result in performance degradation on any job he is able to find. At this point, the vicious circle comes into play: acute POSR causes substandard job performance with the possibility of being fired coupled with family hardship, all resulting in a further increase in the intensity of POSR, still poorer on-the-job performance, and so on around the circle (see above). However, with the help of a financial adviser, a low-interest home equity loan is negotiated, all bills are paid, and the home mortgage payment reduced significantly. In sum, the financial counselor (A in ABC) had suggested a set of contingencies which our hypothetical debtor "saw" as possible PRC's and ARC's for overcoming the harsh barriers or stressors resulting from his deep indebtedness. He carried out the recommended contingencies (B in ABC), the end result (C in ABC) being the removal of the high-SEP stressors and, at the same time, a significant reduction in the intensity level of POSR. Of course, in order to sustain this compensated adjustment state, satisfactory employment must soon materialize or the processes depicted in the vicious circle will eventually reoccur.

In the present ever-accelerating computer age, it may be well to point out that the planned sequences of activities or contingencies for achieving specific goals (C in ABC), central to the examples of the dynamics of stress cited above, are, in computer language, called algorithms. The specific steps in the algorithm are called feedforward processes. Obviously, the algorithm concept is an essential aspect of the ABC model of stress.

4

Basic Equations Suggested by the ABC Model

A mathematical equation is an expression of the equality of two quantities. On the other hand, a symbolic or discursive equation, often used as a pedagogical device, is a representation of the interaction between or among two or more variables or parameters. Following are a series of the latter type of equations, which are logical extensions of the ABC model of *stress*.

As noted in the front material to this book, in the seventeenth century, the English physicist Sir Robert Hooke published an important principle dealing with the elasticity of metals. Known as Hooke's Law, it states in Latin, "*et tensio, sic vis*," or, translated freely into English, "as the stretching, so is the force." In the language of ratios and proportions, Hooke's equation becomes:

$$\text{Stretching Stress (e.g, a rod, units in cms.)} = K \frac{\text{Applied Force (dynes)}}{\text{Cross-Sectional area (cm}^2\text{)}}$$

where K = the proportionality constant for the type of metal of which the rod is composed.

Analogous to Hooke's equation, a discursive expression pertaining to POSR for humans becomes[148]:

$$POSR_{jr} = K_j \frac{IED_r}{AR_j} \tag{4.1}$$

where,

$POSR_{jr}$ = Patterns of Stress Reacitvity for person "j" in situation "r."
IED_r = Intensity of Environmental Demands in situation "r."
AR_j = Adaptive resources of person "j."
K_j = proportionality constant for person "j."

In statement form, Equation 4.1 becomes: the intensity and perhaps the specific characteristics of the POSR are directly proportionate to the IED imposed in situation "r" and inversely proportionate to the AR of person "j" in that situation, the interrelationship being moderated by "K_j," the proportionality constant for "j." "K_j," in turn, is defined by the interaction of so-called moderator variables, variables such as age and gender that may affect the relationship between POSR and the IED/AR ratio in Equation 4.1. From Equation 4.1, an expanded definition of *stress* (POSR) consists of the total organismic reactivity of a person in an environmental situation or set of circumstances in which IED significantly exceeds the AR of that person, taking into account the moderating effect of "K." Although the relationship is not linear in most instances, it is hypothesized that the intensity of POSR is at least a monotonic function of the degree to which IED exceeds AR. An applied example of this definition of *stress* comes from the literature of nuclear submarines: significant POSR (tension, breathing and heart rate increases, headaches) occur for the majority of the crew when the concentration of carbon dioxide (CO_2) in the ambient atmosphere of the deeply submerged "sub," normally at 0.03 percent on the surface with the hatches open, reaches 1.2 percent or higher for a duration of 2–3 hours. Roughly, 0.5 percent exposure to CO_2 is considered the maximum allowable concentration of this toxic gas.

Examples of moderator variables (K_j in Equation 4.1) with respect to which individuals differ greatly, are: age, sex, educational achievement level, general health status, amount and kind of experience in stressful environments, and certain personality trait configurations.

The concept "Intensity of Environmental Demands," IED_r in Equation 4.1, refers to the synergistic effect of the major stressors impinging upon a person "j" at a given time in a specified environment, "r." Stressors differ in terms of their capacity to evoke significant POSR in certain environmental circumstances, that is, they differ in terms of their SEP. For example, excessive heat as compared to a cantankerous supervisor in the same setting would quite likely differ sharply in terms of their SEP's for most people. Thus, equation 4.2 becomes:

$$IED_{jr} = SEP_{\text{Stressor I}} + SEP_{\text{Stressor II}} + \ldots SEP_{\text{Stressor k}} \qquad (4.2)$$

In statement form, Equation 4.2 becomes: The IED for person "j" in environmental situation "r" equals the sum of the SEP of Stressor $_{I}$ plus the SEP of Stressor $_{II}$ and so on through the "k'th" Stressor[145]. The units for the SEP of each stressor are normalized standard scores calculated from the percentile ranks obtained from a person's rank ordering of the self-judged SEP of the major stressors in his/her environment in a stated time interval. In the nuclear submarine service, this technique involving each submariner's rank ordering of the self-perceived stressors in the submerged submarine was called the SIRO (Stressor Identification and Rank Ordering) technique. The SIRO technique provided a useful index of the IED of submariners who were required to adapt for long periods of time to the unique and indeed very high-SEP stressors of the deeply submerged submarine. The SIRO technique, with examples of its application, will be discussed in Chapters 8 and 9.

Equation 4.1 indicates that in order to estimate the POSR for a given person (in addition to estimating IED by SIRO), it is also necessary to estimate that person's AR, the denominator of Equation 4.1. This measure of AR for a given person is generally normative rather than absolute. Accordingly, the most reliable estimate of AR is the sum of the standard scores for a given person on selected measures of the quality of adaptation obtained from a sample of individuals for whom the POSR data are being sought. Some of the measures used with nuclear submariners were: demographic indices, such as age, education and marital status, verbal and mathematical aptitudes, general health status, and the kind and amount of experience with high-SEP stressors[139]. Paired-comparison supervisory ratings and peer ratings on a number of personality trait dimensions, such as emotional stability, affability, and attitudes toward the nuclear submarine service, were also used in some instances to estimate the AR of nuclear submariners[133, 139].

Although some of the variables affecting the intensity of the POSR to a given IED situation are broadly depicted by Equation 4.1, the ABC model suggests additional concepts intrinsically related to the dynamics of stress, that is, processes involved in the opposition of the forces of goal-directed contingencies encountering environmental impediments or barriers of varying degrees of permeability (B_I and B_{II} in Figure 2.1). Equation 4.3 presents some of the factors that tend to affect the intensity of POSR[145].

POSR = (f) A. Effect of "mods"
B. IED/AR ratio
C. Expectancy of Outcome Ratio, $RF^{\pm}/Pu^{\pm}$
D. Valence of Goals or Outcomes
E. Clarity of PRC's and ARC's (4.3)

Assuming that the moderator variables or "mods" (A in Equation 4.3) are relatively constant, Equation 4.3 suggests that the intensity of POSR tends to be elevated for a person for whom "B" was high, "C" was low, most goals in "D" had negative or zero valence, and "E" was low or obscure. More specifically, considering Equation 4.1 and Equation 4.3 together, a significant increase in the IED/AR ratio as the result of heightened IED and/or a deficiency in AR would result in an increase in POSR. Moreover, a similar effect would occur if a person's "expectancy" (subjective probability) that the Outcome Ratio ($RF^{\pm}/Pu^{\pm}$) would decrease significantly as a result of low expectancy of meaningful $RF^{\pm}$ and/or a high expectancy of elevated $Pu^{\pm}$. Also, POSR would tend to increase if few or no goals or outcomes had positive valence and/or if a number of goals had zero or negative valence (see Glossary). Finally, if no contingencies for positive or negative goals are apparent (PRC's) or can be expected to appear in the future (ARC's), that is, the person has no means by which strong NPP's can be satisfied, POSR may be expected to intensify.

Examples of the processes tending to contribute to the intensification of POSR abound. Submariners at 1000 feet depth with insufficient compressed air to blow water ballast to allow the Archimedes buoyancy principle to effect a surfacing of the submarine is an example of this "no win" situation[141]. The archives of the submarine service attest to the fact that very high POSR prevail for the majority of the crew under these circumstances, or, as mentioned earlier, the occupational obsolescence of the late middle-aged executive facing mandatory retirement, a terminally ill person with intense, intractable pain, or a soldier in a foxhole surrounded by the enemy all serve as realistic examples of POSR-intensifying situations involving the dynamisms contained in Equation 4.3.

5
Classification of Stressors Based on the ABC Model

Stressors are aspects of the environment (persons, places, or things) that function as impediments or barriers to goal-directed activity, and, as a result, cause various degrees of emotional reactivity or POSR (see Figure 2.1)[138, 148]. In general, elevated POSR, that is, *stress*, acute or chronic, results from exposure to stressors of varying degrees of SEP. Already mentioned as one method for estimating the SEP of an array of stressors is the SIRO technique involving the Q-sorting procedure described in the Glossary. Two assumptions underpin SIRO: first, that appropriately motivated persons can and will identify many, perhaps most, of the major stressors in their environment at a specified time, and, second, that the same raters can meaningfully rank order this array of stressors by Q-sorting them according to their relative SEP's. For example, studies involving SIRO were conducted in the 1950's and 1960's by several samples of nuclear submariners[134]. These studies yielded a list of stressors characteristic of the environment of the nuclear submarine. In descending order of SEP, these were: perceived danger of radiation and other atmospheric contaminants, concern about seawater pressurization, space restriction, family separation, adverse effects of asynchrony of day-night cues upon sleep, excessive noise levels, work overload and underload, and environmental conditions tending to produce insomnia, boredom, and fatigue.

Table 5.1 contains a partial list of more universal stressors, each with an estimate of SEP, clarity of PRC's and ARC's, expectancy or OR (Outcome Ratio), and lifeline periods during which IED is maximum.

It should be clearly stated at the outset that the estimates of PRC's and ARC's, expectancy or outcome ratios, and IED intensities presented in Table 5.1 are exactly that, estimates based upon inferences from the literature of nuclear submarines, and from survey and review texts on *stress*[20, 25, 56]. Moreover, the

Table 5.1
Classification of Stressors Based upon the ABC Model

Classes of Stressors	SEP[a] Lo-----Hi	Clarity of PRC[b]/ARC[c] Lo-----Hi	Expectancy[d] ratio Lo-----Hi	Period(s) of Lifeline with Highest IED[e]: Childhood Early	Childhood Late	Adolescence Early	Adolescence Late	Adulthood Early	Adulthood Late	Advanced Age Early	Advanced Age Late
A. Primary Stressors											
1. Deprivation: Food, water, clean air, waste elimination, housing	X	X	X	X	X	X	X	X	X	X	X
2. Threats to survival: Heat, cold, noise, natural catastrophes, crowding	X	X	X	X	X				X	X	X
3. Organic dysfunction: Pain, incapacitation, sensory deficiencies	X	X	X X	X	X				X	X	X
B. Secondary Stressors											
1. Barriers to skills development	X	X	X	X	X	X	X	X			
2. Role model absent or obscure	X	X	X	X	X	X	X	X			
3. Threats to Ego/Self esteem	X	X	X		X	X	X	X			
4. Independence/dependence conflict	X	X	X			X	X	X			X
5. Conflicting Social Norms	X	X	X		X	X	X	X			
6. Role ambiguity/role conflict	X	X	X		X	X	X	X			
7. Barriers to group entry & status		X	X		X		X	X			
8. Conflict re: occupational choice		X	X	X			X	X			
9. Obscure career pathway	X	X	X				X	X			
10. Family responsibilities	X	X	X				X	X			
11. Barriers to job advancement	X	X	X						X		
12. Loss of social supports	X	X	X						X	X	X
13. Unattainability of Achievement goals	X	X	X						X	X	
14. Degradation of vital capacity	X	X	X						X	X	X
15. Occupational obsolescence	X	X	X						X	X	
16. Work overload/work underload		X	X	X					X	X	
17. "Empty nest" situation		X	X	X					X	X	
18. Mandatory retirement		X	X	X					X		
19. Catastrophic illness	X	X	X							X	X
20. Degradation of Self-concept	X	X	X						X	X	X

[a]SEP = Stress evocation Potential; [b]PRC = Perceived Reinforcement Contingency; [c]ARC = Anticipated Reinforcement Contingency; [d]Expectancy ratio = ratio of $RF^{\pm}/Pu^{\pm}$, where $RF^{\pm}$ = plus and minus reinforcement and $Pu^{\pm}$ = plus and minus punishment; [e]IED = Intensity of Environmental Demands.

classes of stressors originating from the same sources are not meant to be a complete tabulation, but rather a partial list of the major types of stressors described in the vast literature of this field.

Similarly, the estimated SEP for a given class of stressor is an inference from the same literature and denotes the likelihood that exposure to this type of stressor will result in significant POSR. For example, although less likely to occur in the populations of the industrial West, chronically elevated POSR resulting from such primary stressors as food and water deprivation are the rule rather than the exception for many of the Third World countries of the Middle and Far East.

The basis for the broad classification of stressors as "primary or secondary" in Table 5.1 should be explained. Appearing in the literature of nuclear submarines, this classification coincides with the categorization of needs as primary or secondary. Primary and secondary needs may be differentiated as follows: *primary needs* are unlearned, are cyclic in intensity, and their satisfaction is vital for survival; whereas *secondary needs* are learned, are noncyclic, and their satisfaction is nonvital. Thus, if a motivational vector, underpinned by a primary need (the need for oxygen, for example) is blocked or impeded by the absence or insufficiency of oxygen, then the stressor is *primary*. Similarly, if a secondary need (need for affiliation, for instance) is the most elevated need in the NPP (Figure 3.1) in a given circumstance and the preferred reinforcement contingency(ies) is/are obstructed by an environmental situation resulting in social isolation, the class of stressor involved is labeled *secondary*[138].

Clarity of PRC's and ARC's, column 3 in Table 5.1, refers to the degree to which appropriate contingencies for a predominant need in the NPP are perceived to exist at the time a given set of high-SEP stressors are encountered or are anticipated to be imposed sometime in the future. The PRC's and ARC's and the subsequent contingencies selected to resolve the role ambiguity or role conflict associated with a new job in a poorly structured organization would be a fairly typical example of such a situation[103].

Obviously, the Expectancy or OR in column 4 in Table 5.1 is highly correlated with the ratings of "Clarity of PRC's and ARC's" in column 3. This is true because the expectancy or subjective probability that the ratio of $RF\pm/Pu\pm$, the OR, will be maximized is dependent upon the perceived presence of adequate contingencies for the attainment of the goal or goals appropriate for the existing NPP. Having failed the comprehensive examination, a doctoral aspirant would probably sustain a low OR because, in reality, there are few, if any, immediate PRC's or ARC's expedient for being admitted to another doctoral program for a student with this academic history.

The identification of points on one's lifeline at which the IED tends to be elevated as the result of the imposition of high-SEP stressors is an important consideration from the standpoint of stress prophylaxis, a topic to be addressed in Chapter 8. The content of Table 5.1 suggests, for example, that the most severe IED for the child results from stressors related to skills development, ego or self-esteem formation, role identification, and other socialization processes.

On the other hand, for the adolescent, stressors related to the "dependence/independence" and norm-compliance conflicts largely account for the elevated IED during this period[59, 71]. For the early adult, stressors such as occupational preparation and choice, career pathway establishment, and the imposition of family responsibilities tend to raise the IED during this time span[75].

Finally, stressors related to career plateauing, occupational obsolescence, frustration of achievement goals, loss of vital capacity, removal of social support systems, forced retirement, and illness may result in intense IED during the late adult and advanced age time frames. In particular, POSR during these periods tend to become quite severe because of significant decrements in the AR component of the IED/AR ratio (Equation 4.1).

In summary, since the lifeline concept used in Table 5.1 implies the relative position of a specific stressor ranked in terms of its SEP in a SIRO, distribution would likely vary between individuals at a given time as well as within individuals over time. Thus, the SEP of old stressors may diminish or, in some cases, increase, and new, high-SEP stressors may be imposed. For instance, stressors associated with career choice in early adulthood may be replaced by stressors related to job security after employment in the late adult time frame. As the result of this variation, to be effective, particularly for persons with chronically elevated POSR, SIRO or a similar stressor auditing procedure used to identify major high-SEP stressors should be repeated at intervals usually signaled by significant fluctuation in the intensity of POSR. In sum, the overall conclusion is that the contents and the implications of the information in Table 5.1, while quite useful in understanding POSR, should be construed as being quite tentative and incomplete, requiring further expansion and verification.

6

Acute and Chronic Effects of Stress

The number of classes of processes listed in Table 3.3 attest to the complexity of POSR. As suggested in earlier discussions, the total organismic reactivity pattern called POSR may be characterized as a complex, negative-emotional response pattern similar to that found in depression, anxiety, fear, and anger.

What are the major consequences for the general health status and overall quality of adjustment of a person exposed for a considerable length of time to an array of stressors with high SEP? Figure 6.1 contains some of the possible emotional, behavioral, psychophysiological, and medical conditions that may develop from the acute or chronic POSR caused by exposure to these high-SEP stressors.

To begin with, it is important to note that both the acute and chronic effects of exposure to high-SEP stressors are highly interdependent as indicated by the arrows in Figure 6.1. Acute POSR, usually intense but short-lived, generally occur from the exposure to very high-SEP stressors of short duration, for example, academic or business failure, loss of a loved one, or a natural disaster, such as a fire or a San Francisco earthquake. Hans Selye, in his development of the GAS (General Adaptation Syndrome) model labeled the initial reaction to stressors of this kind as the "alarm" phase, a generalized sympathicotonic fear pattern (see Tables 3.1, 3.2, 3.3, and Figure 6.1) [105, 107]. The alarm phase is usually followed by the "stage of resistance" characterized by the activation of the body's adrenal and other homeostatic systems. Finally, if the person's AR are inadequate, the "exhaustive" phase eventuates and the quality of adaptation may decompensate, a term implying that the intensity of POSR increases at a faster rate than the compensatory or adaptive mechanisms can mobilize. In extreme cases, death from shock may occur during this last phase. On the other hand, if the person's AR are sufficient, the prognosis for the

Figure 6.1
Acute and Chronic Effects of Exposure to High-SEP Stressors

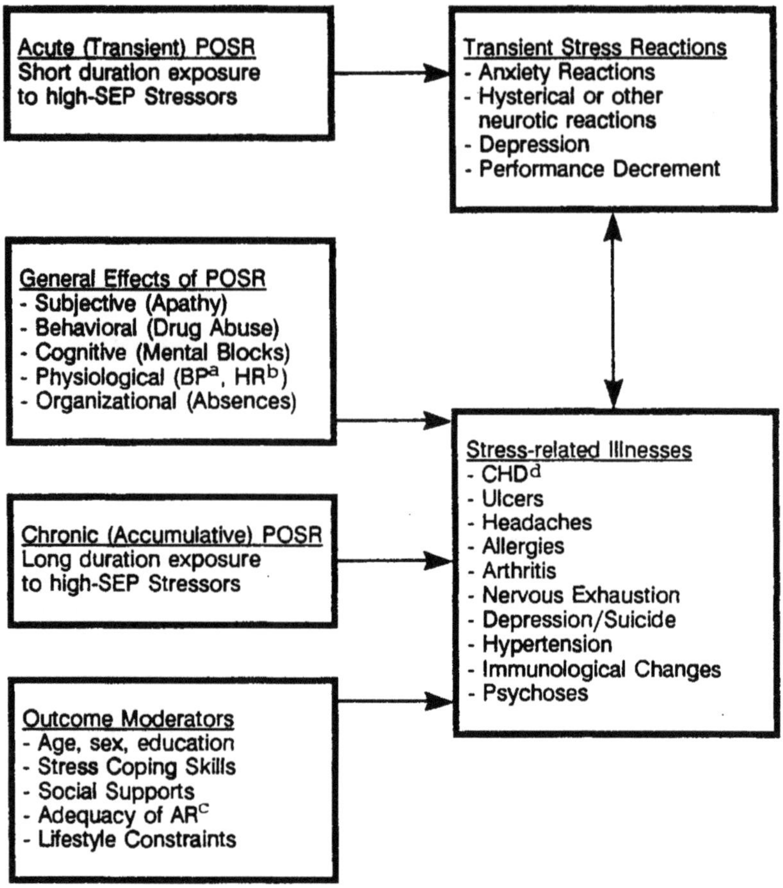

[a]BP—blood presure: [b]HR—heart rate; [c]AR—adaptive resources; [d]CHD—coronary heart disease.

alleviation of acute POSR is quite favorable, much more so than for chronically elevated POSR, which may have persisted for weeks or months.

As stated above, both acute and chronic POSR overlap significantly; however, chronic reactions tend to be more benign at the outset, to be sustained over time, and to occur to low-SEP but more persistent stressors. Moreover, one of the consequences of being subjected to stressors of this kind is that chronically elevated POSR tend to be accumulative, often for extended time intervals. Forty hours weekly in a work setting with a cantankerous supervisor, a turbulent marriage situation, or a progressive illness with increasingly intense and intractable pain are examples of stressor situations likely to result in chronic POSR of considerable intensity. According to Selye[105], the resistance state of GAS is prolonged in these situations, and may be accompanied by accelerated endocrinological and autonomic reactivity. As seen in Figure 6.1, functional and structural changes in a number of organ systems may contribute to coronary heart disease, ulcers, asthma, arthritis, headaches, skin disorders, and so on. Although not empirically documented in many cases, the copious literature of psychosomatic medicine contains numerous suggestions that almost all diseases and injuries have a stress-related component[44].

Recalling the previous discussion of the vicious circle paradigm regarding the cause and effect circularity of stress disorders and illnesses, it seems reasonable, and indeed is partially supported by the literature, that a person's distress from the pain of an ulcer or a migraine headache, for example, may result in the exacerbation of the emotional processes involved (somatopsychic direction), which, in turn, may intensify the correlated somatic processes (psychosomatic direction). This circular process at least partially explains the increases in the rate of organ deterioration and dysfunction as the POSR become chronic.

The renowned Canadian physician Sir William Osler seemed to have recognized this relationship more than a hundred years ago as adjudged by his often cited comment, "It is perhaps as important to know what kind of person has the disease than what kind of disease the person has."

CLASSIFICATION OF STRESS-RELATED ILLNESSES BY THE AMERICAN PSYCHIATRIC ASSOCIATION[29]

Although conceptual and methodological problems of defining mental health and its presumed opposite, mental illness, including stress-related illnesses, have been considerable, some areas of agreement are beginning to appear among the many psychiatrists, psychologists, and social workers active in this field[104]. More and more, the most useful criterion of mental illness appears not only to be related to the incidence and severity of psychopathological symptoms, but also, and perhaps more importantly, to the degree to which these symptoms result in social dysfunctioning or, in extreme cases, social incapacitation[96]. This "social-dysfunctional" criterion of mental health/illness is particularly apropos of the problem of classifying stress-related illnesses, since many of the stressors causing POSR are social in nature (Table 5.1).

The connotation of the "Rumpelstiltskin Fallacy" mentioned in Chapter 1, however, raises the question of the usefulness of the procedure of classifying stress illnesses in the first place. Unlike organic illnesses, (bacterial pneumonia, for example), stress-related conditions, in most cases, have no precisely identifiable pathogen as the sole or even the major etiological agent. Moreover, in the case of a duly diagnosed organic illness, removing the pathogen more often than not cures the illness. This is not the case when dealing with stress-related disorders. In fact, labeling some poorly defined pathological condition (secondary hypertension, for instance) a stress illness may divert the diagnostician away from some obscure, but nevertheless real, organic pathology (kidney disease, for example).

However, legal constraints associated with third party payments of the sky-rocketing costs of medical treatment have forced health care professionals to develop and apply nosological systems to all illnesses, including stress-related illnesses. In 1980, in response to this requirement, the APA (American Psychiatric Association) published the third edition of the *Diagnostic and Statistical Manual of Mental Disorders*, the so-called DSM-III, which contained five-digit codes identifying in detail numerous classes and subclasses of psychiatric disorders. These codes are retained in computer storage and can be easily accessed for the purpose of setting treatment fees and for maintaining continuity between treatment sessions.

The revised edition of DSM-III, DSM-III-R, was published in 1987[29]. One unique feature of DSM-III-R was the so-called multiaxial classification system. The purpose of this system can be most accurately explained by a direct quote from the DSM-III-R manual itself, "DSM-III-R has a multiaxial system for evaluation to ensure that certain information that may be of value in planning treatment and predicting outcome for each person is recorded on each of the five axes. Axes I and II comprise the mental disorders; Axis III, physical disorders and conditions; and Axes IV and V, severity of psychosocial stressors and global assessment of functioning, respectively. In its entirety, the multiaxial system provides a biopsychosocial approach to assessment" (p. 11).

It is seen from the above quotation that Axis IV, "severity of psychosocial stressors," deals directly with the problem of classifying stress disorders. This classification process involves two six-point scales yielding rankings in terms of the "severity of psychosocial stressors," one for adults and another for children and adolescents[29]. For each of the six scale points on the two rating scales, there are anchoring statements or adjectives indicating the severity of the stressors for the person being evaluated: code or rank "1" is "None," whereas codes 2, 3, 4, 5, and 6 are anchored by mild, moderate, severe, extreme, and catastrophic, respectively. In addition, coinciding with each code or scale position are two sets of statements presenting examples of the kinds of stressors that have been rated at a designated level of severity. For instance, for code 2 (mild) on the adult scale in the column headed "acute events" are the statements "Broke up with boyfriend or girlfriend; started or graduated from school; child left home." Also, for the same scale position under a column headed "Enduring circumstances" are the statements: "Family arguments; job dissatisfaction; residence in high crime neighborhood." Time dimensions for the two stressor evaluation columns expanding the severity scales are explicit, namely, "acute events" refers to stressors of less than six months' duration, whereas the column "enduring circumstances" pertains to stressors of greater than six months' duration. Similar anchoring statements, indicating increasingly greater degrees of severity of the stressor situation, coincide with the scale positions 3 to 6. Exactly the same ranking and stressor evaluation format is used for the children and adolescent scales as for the adult scale. In sum, the purpose of the two "Severity of Psychosocial Stressor" scales for Axis IV is to provide a ranking system coded for computer analysis and aimed at assessing the severity of the "psychosocial stressors" that have occurred in the year preceding the differential diagnostic evaluation being conducted.

There is, however, one class of stress disorders not included by APA in the one-year time interval criterion for classification, namely, the so-called PTSD (Post-Traumatic Stress Disorder), which has been assigned the code 309.88. PTSD is characterized by intrusive distressing recollections and recurrent dreams associated with a past "psychologically distressing event that is outside the range of usual human experience, i.e., outside the range of such common experiences as simple bereavement, chronic illness, business losses, and marital conflicts"[29, p. 247ff].

Since the end of the Vietnam War in 1972, PTSD has been diagnosed for a sizeable number of veterans of that engagement. "Generally speaking, these cases have characteristically presented most of the four broad symptoms categories prodromal for PTSD. These are as follows: (1) the traumatic experience was severe, a buddy's corpse, severed, bloody limbs, etc; (2) the traumatic event is persistently reexperienced; (3) strong motivation to avoid any stimuli associated with the event; and (4) persistently high arousal level affecting the quality and quantity of sleep, hypervigilance and explosive outbursts of anger" (ibid).

Since PTSD generally has strong emotional components, mainly anxiety and depression, the standard treatment for this syndrome is similar to that employed for most nonpsychotic emotional disorders. Some of the major treatment modalities used for this kind of disorder will be discussed in the treatment section in Chapter 8.

7

The Assessment of Individual Differences in SCC (Stress Coping Capacity)

Stress Coping Capacity, or SCC, is defined in the Glossary as "an index purported to measure individual differences in a person's ability to adapt adequately to a specified set of stressors." Looking at the equation POSR = K(IED/AR), it appears logical that SCC is some complex function of the reciprocal of Equation 4.1. Thus the equation becomes

$$SCC = K(AR/IED) \tag{7.1}$$

Stated verbally, SCC is directly proportional to AR and inversely proportional to IED. "K," the proportionality constant, which includes a number of moderator variables, similarly tends to take on reciprocal properties. For example, educational achievement level, a moderator variable, is assumed to be negatively correlated with the intensity of POSR but positively correlated with SCC. In general, therefore, the several approaches for the enhancement of SCC to be discussed in this chapter are focused, in one way or another, upon the interrelationships of the variables depicted in Equation 7.1.

SCC ESTIMATED FROM PAIN/DISCOMFORT TOLERANCE TESTS

Originating in the U.S. Marine Corps during World War II, the term "SNAFU tolerance" was used to describe the duration and/or intensity of battlefront conditions a marine could or would withstand before a debilitating breakdown occurred. G. L. Freeman's term PPM, "Psychiatric Plimsoll Mark," has about the same connotation, that is, the maximum stressor intensity (IED) and/or length of exposure required to produce significant psychopathological symptoms in a sizable number of persons involved[38]. For nuclear submariners, with normal shore-based levels of carbon dioxide (CO_2) at 0.03 percent, the length of exposure to the ambient atmosphere of a submerged submarine at 1 percent CO_2 before severe headaches and other symptoms occur in at least 50 percent of the crew is a specific example of the application of the same concept[140]. This index used in the submarine service is called SAD_{50} (Significant Adaptive Decrement in 50 percent of the crew). SAD_{50} is analogous to LD_{50}, the lethal dosage of a specified pharmaceutical agent for 50 percent of a specified animal sample.

Therefore, one possible approach to estimating a person's SCC is to measure the intensity and/or duration of exposure to selected environmental stressors sufficient to cause significant decompensation in his/her quality of adjustment in a given circumstance and at a given time. Reviewing the basic Equation 4.1, POSR = K[IED/AR], it is seen that these three indexes of individual differences in SCC, SNAFU tolerance, Psychiatric Plimsoll, and SAD_{50}, have a common denominator; namely, they are all threshold indices indicating the maximum IED that a person can (will?) withstand before significant maladaptive trends develop, assuming of course that K and AR are held constant.

In practice, what methods can be used to estimate individual differences in these threshold measures? More specifically, how can the intensity of IED be increased sufficiently to produce maladaptive signs or symptoms sufficiently severe to suggest a reliable estimate of SCC? What about the ethics of this procedure? A German submarine officer was selected during World War II by measuring how much electrical current delivered to the palm of his hand the candidate could or would withstand before he said "enough." Similarly, this technique of measuring the pain, discomfort, or distress tolerance has also been used by the U.S. military, for example, the stress interview used by the OSS (Office of Strategic Services) and the merciless training routine that the aggressive marine drill sergeant forces the marine "boot" to endure. The medically dangerous "forced urinary retention" technique and the grueling outdoor training of adolescents enrolled in the "Outreach Program" are other examples of similar procedures used with civilian groups to produce elevated IED situations[39]. Although there is a persistent public attitude that demonstrated ability to withstand pain and discomfort correlates positively with SCC, there is no substantive empirical data to support this contention.

The fact that measures of individual differences in pain/discomfort tolerance in contrived high-SEP situations have only very low correlation with differences in SCC in real life can be explained in part rather simply: the contrived high-IED situation involves a rather narrow range of stressors, namely, those causing pain and discomfort. On the other hand, real-life situations are much more complex, and are associated with an array of stressors varying from pain and discomfort to socially imposed impediments to career development and job security (*see* Table 5.1).

SCC ESTIMATED FROM SIMULATOR PERFORMANCE

To correct this discrepancy between contrived and real-life IED situations, the era of computerized simulation was ushered in during the early 1960's. Attempting to replicate the "real" environmental conditions of concern, these simulators began to appear both in the military and civilian sectors, for example, the Link Trainer for aviators, the attack, mooring and docking, and fire control simulators for submariners, and the weightlessness and high-gravity centrifuge simulators for astronauts. Data obtained from judgments made by trained observers of the person's performance in the simulator together with objective measures of the performance itself (psychophysiological measures, reaction time, error counts, and so on) provide the basis for estimating individual differences in SCC[127].

As before, the same question arises: Are these data collected during simulator performance usefully valid predictors of SCC in real life? One way to enhance the validity of this relationship is to improve the quality of the simulation. A great deal of research has gone into improving what simulation experts call the "ecological representativeness" of simulated environments. This research has produced the dual concepts of *physical fidelity* and *psychological fidelity*, the latter, a new concept, meaning the extent to which the psychological components (prevailing IED, interpersonal relationships, and so on) in the simulated situation "A" are similar to those in "B," the real-life situation. In general, it appears that adequate psychological fidelity can occur between environments with rather low physical fidelity (spatial constraints, ambient atmosphere, and the like)[127].

Much of the published literature pertaining to the fidelity of simulation comes from the military and aerospace industries. For instance, one study conducted during the Korean War involved the correlation of observational data of infantrymen performing in a simulated battlefield at an army base in the United States with the dichotomous criterion did/did not panic (the so-called "freeze" reaction) on the Korean battlefield[8]. In general, there was no systematic relationship between the two data bases. Slightly more optimistic were the low but nonchance correlations between submarine and aerospace simulator data and performance under actual space flight or submerged conditions. In short, the basic assumption underlying the continued use of simulators seems to be supported: "if a person shows sufficiently severe POSR to result in significant performance degradation during the relatively low-IED conditions maintained during simulation, it is highly unlikely that this same person can adapt adequately to the high-IED conditions characteristically found in the real-life exposure to a variety of high-SEP stressors" [139].

SCC ESTIMATED FROM AR (ADAPTIVE RESOURCES)

Up to this point, the focus on the problem of estimating SCC has been on the numerator of Equation 4.1, that is, upon the intensity of POSR resulting from extreme IED situations. Another approach to the same problem would be to estimate a person's SCC by focusing upon the denominator of Equation 4.1, namely AR, the hypothesis being that the greater the AR, the less intense the POSR and, by inference, the greater the SCC.

Biographical Data

It is almost a truism that one of the most valid predictors of *future* behavior is *past* behavior. On the surface, it seems reasonable that appropriately collected biodata, as it has come to be called (information pertaining to the quality of the adjustment of a person to past high-IED situations) should be a useful source of data for predicting his/her SCC for similar circumstances in the future[143].

With an almost unlimited array of biographical information available, however, which items of biodata have the highest validity for this purpose? First, items from the person's medical record, especially the psychiatric history during the developmental years, may be related to his/her AR. Examples of these biodata are: disease history, incidences of hospitalization, treatment for mental illness, and so forth. Also, information regarding educational achievement, interests, values, and attitudes may similarly be useful in assessing a person's AR. History of exposure to high-IED situations (for example, family bereavement, injuries or illness, academic or occupational impediments, and even failure) and data pertaining to overall quality of social adjustment, such as delinquency and criminal records, may also contribute to an evaluation of a person's AR. It should be recalled in this context that Table 5.1 contains a compilation of stressor categories, many of which may be used as criteria with respect to which a person's past adjustment history may be evaluated. With submariners, multitrait rating paired comparison scales (adaptability, frustration tolerance, and so on), completed by expert observers familiar with the performance of the rating specialties as well as with the IED of the submarine environment itself, have been used to assess the AR of the nuclear submarine recruit[129, 130, 134].

Ability Test Data

Dating as far back as the 1920's, the literature dealing with functional intelligence as measured mainly by IQ tests, has supported the general proposition that persons with above average to superior intelligence tend to be healthier, both mentally and physically, to attain higher educational achievement levels, and to be more adequately adjusted overall than less intelligent person[115]. Recalling the ABC model (Figure 3.1) and Equation 4.1, it is seen that the intensity of POSR is inversely proportional to AR. The logical implication follows that AR is related to the effectiveness of the contingencies available for a person's overcoming or circumventing environmental barriers to goal-directed behavior. In turn, therefore, the AR and hence the SCC of the more intelligent segment of the population would be expected to be greater, since they are able to learn more effective ways (PRC's and ARC's) to avoid, penetrate, or circumvent barriers (stressors). The net outcome is that these persons typically experience less severe POSR to extreme IED levels and, as a consequence, their SCC is thereby enhanced.

However, a *caveat* should be inserted at this point. If, as the summary statement above implies, measures of ability are correlated with SCC, then prediction of individual difference in the quality of adaptation to high-SEP stressors from ability test scores should be a real possibility. Ability tests, including aptitude and achievement tests, however, do not measure *capacity* directly, but rather they measure differences in *performance* on the specific items making up the test or other measures of abilities. Even trained test administrators somewhat naively assume that the person being tested is maximally cooperative and is exerting as much effort as possible while being tested. Submariners use the term "will do/can do" ratio to describe this dilemma. Accordingly, as a submariner's will do/can do ratio approaches 100 percent, it may be assumed that this person is maximally motivated to perform close to the limits of his capacity. This difference between what a person will do and what he/she can do, in psychometric parlance, is quite likely a significant source of what is called error variance found in all ability test scores. In part as the result of this source of error, the predictive relationship between ability test scores and SCC is somewhat tenuous at best.

This tenuousness of the relationship between ability test scores and SCC is demonstrated by the suggestive but marginally significant results from several submarine studies. The criterion used in most of these studies is a dichotomous one: qualify or fail to qualify at sea after graduating from submarine school. For instance, scores on the General Classification Test, a measure of verbal aptitude, an arithmetical aptitude test, and a mechanical aptitude test, all yield low, but significant correlation coefficients with the criterion fail to qualify to wear the dolphins, the prestigious symbol of the submarine service[152]. These low to moderate correlational statistics argue strongly that individual differences in the AR and, by extension, the SCC of submariners are multifaceted, with ability differences being only a small part of the total predictive relationship.

Personality Variables

The term "personality" may be defined as "the particular pattern of traits, the structural and functional units of personality, describing a person's unique adjustment to his or her environment"[3]. Roughly equivalent to the lay use of the term "life-style," personality may be operationally defined by a profile of descriptive traits or characteristics quite accurately measured by modern personality tests and observational techniques[47].

There is a growing literature demonstrating the correlation of scores on selected personality tests with SCC. By inference then, the AR and hence the SCC tend to be enhanced for persons: (a) whose scores indicate greater introversive than extroversive tendencies[24], (b) whose "locus of control" tends to be "internal" rather than "external,"[24, 91] (c) who have high levels of self-esteem[86], (d) who display a high "need for achievement"[78], and (e) whose life-style fits more closely the Type B rather than the Type A behavioral pattern[40]. It is interesting as well as informative to note that the above correlation between SCC and *internal* "locus of control" (*see* Glossary) is consistent with the ABC model. That is, the life-style of "internalizers" is based upon the assumption that high-valent outcomes or rewards ("C" in ABC) are, for the most part, contingent on one's own actions ("B" in ABC). These behavioral activities are called PRC's in the model.

The relationship between personality test data and the SCC of nuclear submariners during protracted submerged missions is not at all clear. Neurotic tendencies measured by objective tests bear a low, but nonchance negative relationship with submariner adaptability and performance[146]. In contrast, a positive correlation with SCC holds for an objective measure of motivational intensity and a measure of favorable attitudes toward the submarine service[139, 149]. Further, responses to the color stimuli on the Rorschach Inkblot test also show a low negative correlation with supervisory ratings of SCC[150]. Finally, data obtained from a sentence completion measure of depression proneness, although not formally validated, did show some suggestive relationships to the performance and overall SCC of U.S. Navy divers[141] (*see* Appendix D).

As with the relationship between ability test scores and SCC, a related, but slightly different *caveat* is in order for the correlation between objective personality test scores and SCC. Ability test items, such as arithmetic or mechanical problems, are constructed so as to require the respondent's best or *correct* response or solution in order that these responses can be scored dichotomously, right or wrong, correct or incorrect. On the other hand, personality test items do not require the respondent's *correct* response, but rather his/her most *truthful* response. That is, the person taking the personality test is required to indicate the degree to which such a statement as "I tend to be a nervous person" applies, or is characteristic of himself or herself typically or most of the time. It is a well-documented fact that many respondents to these threatening types of personality test items tend to deny or suppress admissions that make them look "bad." Instead, there is a strong tendency to give socially desirable responses, that is, responses that make them look "good" or those that they think the test administrator wants them to give. Thus, some of the error variance attenuating the reliability of the relationship between scores on an objective personality test and SCC depends upon the degree to which the testee is "open"—uninhibited and willing to cooperate and respond as honestly as possible to items whose content is often personal and private, possibly embarrassing, and sometimes, downright threatening, such as, "My sex life is unsatisfactory."

Psychophysiological Indexes

Returning again to the basic Equation 4.1, the ABC model (Figure 3.1), and Tables 3.1, 3.2, and 3.3, it is seen that the patterning of psychophysiological processes constitutes an important component of POSR. At this point, it seems necessary to reiterate that one of the central elements of POSR is emotional in nature, negative emotions in most cases. The major mechanisms of this emotional component involve the ANS and the endocrine system (Tables 3.1, 3.2, and 3.3).

H. Funkenstein, S. H. King, and M. E. Doolette contrasted the so-called epinephrine or anger-directed-out personality type with the norepinephrine or anger-directed-in response type. Although lacking in firm empirical validation, persons typically showing the epinephrine (anger-out) response pattern to a given set of stressors would be most likely to have the greatest SCC[43].

A considerable amount of data dealing with individual differences in ANS function have emerged from submarine and other military research over the past three decades[128, 137, 144]. Overall, the essential concept seems to be "ANS resiliency." Based upon peripheral indexes of ANS function (blood pressure, heart rate, electrical conductance of the skin), differences in the capacity of these indicators to revert to baseline levels following exposure to real or contrived high-IED conditions appear to be useful measures of SCC[137].

Global Trait Ratings

For more than four decades, there has been an ongoing disagreement in the personality assessment field as to whether the intuitive or clinical judgment approach typically used by psychiatrists, clinical psychologists, and social workers is more or less valid for predicting a person's future behavior than is the more complex statistical approach[82]. In spite of the preponderance of evidence tending to favor some type of statistical approach to this predictive problem, claims for the predictive validity of impressionistic judgments still persist.

One version of a global trait rating method was used in the 1960's by interviewers assigned the responsibility of predicting the success of recruits for the nuclear submarine service. A slightly modified version of that rating system was recently published for use by interviewers for screening civilian job applicants[143]. Although substantive validation data for this method do not exist at this time, this multitrait rating technique, labeled GTPSS (Global Trait Psychological Screening System) is nonetheless presented here as a model to be used experimentally as an approach for estimating individual differences in SCC.

The procedure for implementing the GTPSS method is straightforward. The interviewer first conducts an individual interview, adhering as closely as possible to a structured format or an interview schedule, constructed specifically as a companion to the GTPSS. Then, based upon these interview data, which preferably had been recorded, the interviewer circles a number varying from −4 to +4 on each of the nine scales, that number to correspond to his/her considered judgment as to the interviewee's most accurate rating on each dimension. Finally, an AAPS (Applicant's Adjustment Potential Score) (Figure 7.1), considered for

Figure 7.1
Global Trait Rating System

	1	2	3	4	5	6	7	8	9
									AAPS[a]
	+4	+4	+4	+4	+4	+4	+4	+4	+4
Extremely Favorable									
	+3	+3	+3	+3	+3	+3	+3	+3	+3
Somewhat Favorable									
	+2	+2	+2	+2	+2	+2	+2	+2	+2
Slightly Favorable									
	+1	+1	+1	+1	+1	+1	+1	+1	+1
Neither Favorable Nor Unfavorable	0	0	0	0	0	0	0	0	0
	-1	-1	-1	-1	-1	-1	-1	-1	-1
Slightly Unfavorable									
	-2	-2	-2	-2	-2	-2	-2	-2	-2
Somewhat Unfavorable									
	-3	-3	-3	-3	-3	-3	-3	-3	-3
Extremely Unfavorable									
	-4	-4	-4	-4	-4	-4	-4	-4	-4
Scale Ratings	---	---	---	---	---	---	---	---	---

1. General Ability/Aptitude/Achievement: IQ test scores; Educational achievement level and quality (e.g. grades); Other indices of achievement
2. Biographical Data/Developmental History: Family/cultural background; Childhood neuropathic traits and other medical history; Marital and job history (if appropriate) etc.
3. Motivation for the Job: Reasons for wanting the job; Appropriateness of goals--clarity of goal structure; Mode-to-goal orientation; Motivational test scores, etc.
4. Appropriateness and Intensity of Attitudes: Attitudes toward: the work ethic in general, society's rules and regulations; authority in general; rigid social prejudices, etc.
5. Character or Behavioral Traits: Evidence for, or absence of maladaptive trait development; Psychopathic or dyssocial trends; Personality trait or pattern disturbances, etc.
6. Social Trait Patterns: General social adaptability; Communication and other social skills, etc.
7. Frequency and Severity of Neurotic Symptoms: Scores on psychodiagnostic test(s); Characteristic ego defense strategies, etc.
8. Frequency and Severity of Neurotic Symptoms: General orientation and reality contact; Appropriateness of affect; Motor or perceptual functioning, etc.
9. Overall Adjustment Potential: applicant's overall potential for the job.

[a] AAPS: Applicant's Adjustment Potential Score

Source: Reference 143, p. 147. Reprinted by permission of Thieme Inc.

our present purposes to be equivalent to an SCC score, is calculated by algebraically summing the ratings across the nine scales.

To repeat, this rating method has never been appropriately validated but, in spite of this fact, may serve a heuristic function by stimulating systematic research aimed at demonstrating the validity (or lack thereof) of the GTPSS for estimating a person's SCC.

SCC ESTIMATED FROM MODERATOR VARIABLES

Looking again at Equation 4.1, it is seen that the intensity and perhaps the particular characteristics of the POSR are directly related to a class of variables called moderators (mods)[98] (*see* Glossary). The following listing of "mods" is not meant to be complete, but rather to provide a brief evaluation of the most obvious variables significantly affecting the relationship among POSR, IED, and AR.

Age

Inevitably, the aging process involves loss of vital capacity, "*elan vital*," as the French would say. Sensory deficiencies and performance degradation are unavoidable consequences of aging[105]. Since the aging person's AR are limited, it seems reasonable, and indeed the facts tend to provide ample evidence that such stressors as excessive noise, heat, cold, frustration, conflict and loss of social supports generally result in significantly reduced SCC, particularly during advanced age (see Table 5.1).

Gender

The endocrinological, physiological, morphological, and biosocial differences between the sexes are well known. Less well understood are the differences and similarities in the roles of men and women, particularly in the work place. The stressors associated with the persistent tendency for sex role stereotyping have at times and under certain conditions caused severe POSR for both sexes, but more so for women. Sexual harassment and even abuse of women, in both the work and home environment, appear to contribute significantly to a sustained high level of POSR, particularly for those with inadequate AR[20].

Although the argument is somewhat circular in that it is assumed but not proven that POSR have some causal relationship to health deficiencies, men overall have lower life expectancy, are more likely to die of coronary heart disease and alcohol-related illness, have higher accident rates, and have higher suicide rates than women. Some gerontologists argue that one major cause of these sex differences is the relative inadequacy of the SCC of men as compared to women. In short, gender appears to be a significant moderator, and, as a result, should be taken into account when attempting to predict individual differences in the SCC of both men and women.

Educational Achievement Level

In the nuclear submarine service, five categories of this moderator variable were considered important: less than high school, HS dropouts, HS graduate, some college, and finally, college graduate[62]. The educational achievement moderator affects the positive correlation between verbal, mathematical and mechanical aptitude test scores, and rated performance during submarine missions[140, 145]. HS dropouts, even with above average aptitude test scores, have very low probability for success in "subs." Conversely, those recruits who have a HS diploma have a high probability of succeeding irrespective of their test scores. Similar results have been found for submariners who do and do not have a history of drug abuse. That is, past drug abuse history is found disproportionately more frequently in the HS-drop segment than in the HS graduate group. From the standpoint of *stress*, these findings suggest that both poor academic performance and drug abuse by submariners may both be concomitants of chronically elevated POSR, an assumption that seems plausible based upon the data presently available.

Other evidence tending to support the moderating effect of educational achievement on POSR level comes from the civilian literature[59]. For example, Hans Selye reported a study showing that the incidence of stress-related illness was lower for those persons whose educational achievement levels exceeded their culturally determined social status[105]. Similarly, a study of a large group of college men conducted by AT&T found that the incidence of heart disease was significantly lower for college men as compared to a comparable group of noncollege men[52].

In conclusion, whereas the causal linkage is complex and the relationship is nonlinear, SCC seems to be positively correlated with the educational achievement level.

Experience with High-SEP Stressors

The time-worn adage "one gets used to hanging if one hangs long enough" may make an important point. The phenomenon of human adaptation in the area of perception and physiology has been studied quite thoroughly. Examples are the dark adaptation of the eye and the homeostatic control of the acid-base level of the blood and urine. Other examples of adaptation to high-SEP stressors, this time at the behavioral level, are adaptation to excessive heat, cold, noise, crowding, noxious odors, and a variety of fear-producing situations.

An apt example of submariners' physiological adaptation to intense sensory stimulation, an olfactory stressor in this case, occurs after four or five hours submergence. The level of adaptation is attested by the fact that the odor of onions or a well-used cigar cannot be detected[136]. With a plentiful supply of fresh water obtained from desalinated seawater available, the crew members can and do shower frequently. But, except for the prevention of skin disorders, submariners need not shower often because body odor is not offensive to the well-adapted nose. This is true because of the so-called Weber's Law, the ratio of the least perceptible stimulus level to the absolute intensity level of the stimulus. As this ratio approaches unity, the intensity of the stimulus required to be discernible likewise increases. Thus, insofar as odor is concerned, it takes a real wallop to be detectible once this sensory modality becomes completely adapted. About halfway through one 80-day submerged mission, the author asked the submariner who occupied the bunk two bunks above in the 4-tier bunk bed to conduct a simple experiment as follows: it was suggested to this volunteer that the next time he showered he do a sequence of tasks. After lathering thoroughly in the hot steamy shower stream, he took three or four deep breaths of the steam to clear the airways, brought his dungarees hanging nearby into the stall and quickly took a few big whiffs of them. In brief, upon completing this sequence, the submariner's 85-decibel yell could be heard throughout the grid-iron-length "sub." The inhaled steam had neutralized the adaptation process. In ABC language, the clearing of the airways had resulted in a significant increase in the SEP of the olfactory stressor, thus producing a brief but intense stress reaction.

Another study at a different behavioral level was conducted by the paratrooper division of the U.S. Air Force. Very briefly, it was clearly demonstrated that these carefully selected paratroopers showed less and less fear, anxiety, and other POSR as they gained more and more experience following a series of simulated parachute "drops"[8].

General Health Status

The direction of causality poses a serious dilemma when considering the relationship between general health status and POSR. That is, does illness cause POSR or vice versa? One series of studies involving the Social Readjustment Scale, which yields LCU ("Life Change Unit") scores, has shown a consistent positive correlation with illness rates in a variety of population samples[53]. Also, LCU scores, consisting of summed ratings of stressors, such as "death in the family," divorce, marriage, loss of job, and so on, correlated positively with the number of sick call visits of enlisted men in the U.S. Navy[53]. Although the mechanisms are far from clear, the direction of these interrelationships is generally assumed to be from the life change event to POSR, then, in turn, POSR to stress-related illness, and finally, in time, to unfavorable general health status.

From another perspective, however, the direction of causality may be reversed; that is, the general health status of a person may affect his/her POSR level directly. Health care providers are well aware that loud noises, bright lights, and similar stressors, particularly if unexpected, are very noxious to hospitalized patients. In other words, unfavorable general health status appears to exacerbate the SEP of environmental stressors that cause very few POSR in healthy persons. Selye's notion of "available adaptive energy," although not well documented, nonetheless suggests a possible mechanism to explain the relationship between general health status and SCC[107]. Although a long extrapolative leap, this correlation between health and intensity and the configuration of POSR may partially explain the considerable literature supporting the general finding of immunological deficiencies in persons chronically exposed to high-IED situations[26].

EXPERIMENTAL TESTS FOR MEASURING SCC

The methodology for measuring human behavior, such as intelligence, interests and values, personality trait patterning, and SCC has become greatly refined since World War II. Validity, or the degree to which a psychometric instrument in fact measures the processes it purports to measure, can be accurately calculated, particularly since the advent of computer technology. The reliability, or the precision with which behavioral processes are being measured by an experimental test or other measurement device, may also be quite precisely estimated. Since Alfred Binet developed the first intelligence test in the first decade of the twentieth century, a fundamental principle of psychometrics has emerged, namely, "a test instrument must first have adequate reliability if it is to have any useful validity for any purpose." Implied in this statement of a basic psychometric principle is the fact that the reliability and validity of any test or measure are empirical matters, depending upon appropriately collected data bearing on these two interrelated requirements[143].

The following experimental tests were developed to predict individual differences in the SCC of nuclear submariners during submerged missions often exceeding eighty days' duration. As will become apparent, these tests vary from one to another in terms of the amount and quality of the data available to support their reliability and validity for this purpose. Nonetheless, they are presented here for heuristic reasons, that is, to suggest new approaches to measuring SCC to be tested and, if need be, modified by students as well as by experts active in the field of stress research.

PIB (Personal Inventory Barometer)

To an extent, one of the most severe components of POSR is anxiety. Although related to phobia, which is associated with a specific environmental object or situation, anxiety is a more diffuse emotion that results from a persistent dread, apprehension, or foreboding concerning the possible occurrence of *future* events or outcomes. In contrast, another emotional component of POSR, guilt, involves concern, regret, or remorse about *past* events. Because of this time-dimension aspect of the two emotions anxiety and guilt, items designed to measure these emotions came to be called, respectively, the futurovertive and retrovertive parts of the array of experimental test items used during the early developmental stages of the PIB. The overt signs of anxiety, guilt, and related emotions are, for the most part, associated with ANS reactivity, some of the symptoms for which are sweating, skin pallor, pupil dilation, and rapid pulse—signs that are in most cases directly observable (see Table 3.2). On the other hand, covert or subjective symptoms of these emotions are generally inferred from the self-reported, subjective impressions of the person experiencing the emotional reactivity (*see* Table 3.3).

The PIB was developed in 1956 for the purpose of measuring these so-called subjective symptoms of anxiety, guilt, ego-strength, hostile attitudes, and similar personality traits in candidates for the nuclear submarine service[156]. The assumption made then, which has since been partially borne out, was that the number and severity of anxiety and related symptoms are inversely correlated with the SCC of submariners during long submerged missions. Modeled somewhat after the well-known MMPI (Minnesota Multiphasic Personality Inventory), the PIB consisted of fifty statements describing common symptoms and signs of mood, guilt, depression, anxiety, and other similar personality traits. Examples of the original PIB items are: "I worry over money and business; I have been afraid of things or people that I know could not hurt me; I certainly feel useless at times," and so on.

Although the PIB is similar in terms of test item content to the MMPI, the Taylor Manifest Anxiety Scale, and other inventories of this kind, the response format of the PIB is in several ways unique. Most personality tests designed to measure self-impressions of one's own emotional reactivity require the simple, dichotomous either/or, true/false, or yes/no response to each item to indicate whether or not a test item, such as "I wish I were happier," either applies or does not apply, or does or does not describe an individual as he/she "sees" himself or herself generally or most of the time. Thus, the test respondent is placed in a similar position to that of the person asked to respond to the question, "When did you stop beating your mother?" In other words, the respondent is assumed guilty unless he/she proves himself or herself not guilty, exactly the opposite of the fundamental principle of jurisprudence, "innocent until proven guilty."

Since it is a well-documented fact that respondents to this type of test item generally tend to deny or suppress unfavorable descriptive statements about themselves, distributions of scores consisting of summed dichotomous responses tend to be sharply skewed in a positive direction. This statistical tendency reflects that relatively few "yes" or "true" responses to this kind of item content occur when this response format is used. In contrast, the "barometer" response format (Appendix A) used by the PIB is based upon the assumption that the majority of the test respondents are, for example, neither "completely anxious" nor "completely anxiety-free," or neither "very guilty" nor "guiltless." Rather, in reality, most people experience different intensities or degrees of anxiety, guilt, and related emotions. Moreover, exploratory data comparing the score distributions of a large sample of submariners using the true/false response format and the same sample, after many weeks, using the "barometer" format with the same test items clearly demonstrated that significantly less denial and suppression of responses to unfavorable item content occurred when the PIB scale was used[156].

The instructions to the respondent being administered the PIB using the "barometer" response format were (*see* Appendix A):

There are 50 statements, more or less descriptive of most people, contained in the test booklet accompanying the answer sheet. Looking at the answer sheet, you will notice a vertical scale extending from "0" at the bottom, close by a statement "not at all like me" to "9" at the top of the scale near the statement, "exactly like me." Notice also that the numerals between "0" and "9," that is, 1 through 8, are also just above and just below the other three statements: "only slightly like me," "somewhat like me," and "considerably like me," in ascending order. Thus, the larger the number the more closely each item statement describes yourself as you "see" yourself, generally, or most of the time. Note that the five statements are each between two scale numerals and *not exactly* at the same level as any number. Your task then is simply to carefully read each descriptive statement, then select from the "0" to "9" scale, the *ONE* whole number (no fractions or decimals please) indicating the degree to which that item "fits" you as you "see" yourself, generally speaking. Finally, write that scale number in the box on the answer sheet corresponding to the item number. There is no time limit, so work at your own speed. Thanks in advance for your cooperation[156].

There are some unique features of the vertical, ten-point response scale called the "barometer" used by the PIB. First of all, during some early exploratory trials of the PIB using the PIB scale placed both horizontally on some and vertically on other answer sheets, it was clearly demonstrated that the scale in the vertical position yielded significantly more reliable summed item scores with the same fifty items as compared to the scores obtained with the scale in the horizontal position. This finding was interpreted to be the result of a culturally determined response set that more of a "thing" is "up" and less is "down." A thermometer, for example, is never hung horizontally.

Another aspect of the response scale to be noted is the placement of the anchor statements for the ten-point scale, "not at all like me," "somewhat like me," and so on, relative to the "0" to "9" number points on the scale. Accordingly, the five anchor statements are placed *between* two scale numbers, thus forcing the respondent to choose *one* scale number just above or just below the "anchor." This feature of the response scale has the effect of forcing the testee to spread out his or her self-ratings, the overall consequence being to increase the variation of the distributions of responses to each item. Thus, in statistical language, the variance of the total summed PIB scores is similarly significantly increased.

Some general findings regarding the PIB as a predictor of individual differences in the SCC of nuclear submariners are: (1) the use of the "barometer" response format, without question, significantly increases the score variability and virtually removes the positive skew characteristic of score distributions using the true/false or other dichotomous formats. Incidentally, the near normal curve describing PIB score distributions tends to support the validity of the psychological over the medical model of stress described in Chapter 1 in that the processes making up POSR are not different in kind (either they are/are not there), but instead are continuous multivariate processes, differing mainly in degrees of intensity; (2) on the average, the means and SDs (standard deviations) of the PIB score distributions are about 116 and 54 in that order; (3) with the test administrations separated by five to eight weeks, the test-retest reliability averages about 0.80; (4) the validity of the PIB is indicated by the fact that 37 percent of those submariner candidates who fail to pass submarine school and become qualified to wear the dolphins receive PIB scores at or above 180 (1.2 SD units above the mean). In comparison, only 11 percent of those who in fact earn the dolphins receive PIB scores equal or greater than the 180 PIB score cutoff point[156].

In summary, the PIB, after rigorous psychometric analysis and many subsequent revisions over the past thirty years, is still part of the psychiatric screening battery for the 4,000 to 6,000 annual input volunteers for the nuclear submarine service. Assuming that the demographics of the volunteer recruits for the submarine service have not changed significantly during this time span, it would appear that the PIB, possibly with some modification of test item content here and there (but at the same time leaving the "barometer" response format essentially intact), will continue to be a useful predictor of individual differences in the SCC of nuclear submariners.

ARI (Affective Response Inventory)

The term "affect," an important component of POSR, refers to the subjective experience associated with exposure to a pattern of high-SEP stressors. Degrees of intensity of affect lie along a subjective continuum extending from unpleasant (negative affect) to pleasant (positive affect). The ARI is a thirty-item, nine-category bipolar adjective rating scale. Examples of the bipolar rating scales defined by paired descriptors (one on each end of the scales) are contained in Appendix B. The respondents are asked to recall a highly stressful incident that occurred in the past and to check a point on each of the thirty scales indicating the intensity of the affect experienced during the specific situation being recalled. The ARI is scored by summing the responses (1–9) to the 16 direct items (high-stress adjective on the 9 end of the scale) to the remaining 14 reversed items (high-stress descriptor at the 1 end), the latter responses having been subtracted from the constant "10." The high- and low-stress ends of the thirty scales had been previously determined from the unanimous agreement of three psychologist-judges. Hypothetically, the higher the ARI scores, the more intense the affective component of POSR[148].

The ARI mean and SD (standard deviation) in a sample of 23 graduate students was 180 and 24, respectively. In an independent study involving ten graduate students, the ARI correlated with scores on an achievement test on the topic of stress 0.64, $P<0.01$. However, in a cross-validation sample of thirteen graduate students, the correlation coefficient failed to reach significance at the 5 percent confidence level.

Another independent study produced some data bearing on the factorial or construct validity of ARI[148]. As the term "factorial" implies, these data were obtained from an Incremental R-technique factor analysis of ARI change-scores before and after sixteen graduate students had been exposed to a contrived stress situation. Eighty-three percent of the variance in change-scores was accounted for by the first bipolar factor labeled "Reactive anxiety/unpleasant affect." The adjectives receiving the highest loadings on this factor were unconfident, miserable, displeased, anxious, and confused.

WAI (Weybrew Activity Inventory)

One consistent finding in the voluminous literature pertaining to the concept of Type A and Type B personalities is that those persons demonstrating strong Type A traits tend to be time-constrained, always in a hurry, and disturbed by delays of any kind[40, 69, 135]. As is immediately apparent upon an examination of the content of the WAI items in Appendix C, these items are designed to tap these kinds of traits. With the frequency rating scale weighted 3, 2, 1 in the same order for "always or almost always," "occasionally" to "never" (weighing reversed for item 15), the WAI score is calculated by summing these weighted responses over the 22 items.

In a sample of twenty-three graduate students, the mean was forty-two and the SD was five raw score units. In an independent pilot study involving thirteen graduate students, the correlation of WAI scores with scores on an achievement test on the subject of stress was 0.26, suggesting a trend. However, this statistic was not significant at the 5 percent level.

In sum, whereas the hypothesis that the WAI or similar tests measuring patterns of traits related to a "sense of urgency" are systematically related to SCC remains tenable, substantive validation data supporting this relationship are lacking at this time.

IC (Incomplete Sentences)

A consistent finding in the literature of stress is that a significant component of POSR is, in most cases, the presence of mild to severe symptoms of clinical depression. It follows, therefore, that persons prone to become depressed in high-stress situations would be expected to have correspondingly low SCC. The test labeled IC (Incomplete Sentences) in Appendix D consists of thirty-five sentence stems. The IC actually was known to the professional staff as the DPSS (Depression Proneness Sentence Stems), the IC label being used to conceal the real purpose of the test from the respondents. The instructions to the submariners to whom it was experimentally administered were simply, "Following are 35 incomplete sentences. We are asking you to complete these sentence stems by writing in the remainder of each stem. We suggest that you write down the first completion that comes to mind. Sentence structure, grammar, and so on are really not important. Remember—the first thing you think of!"

An examination of the sentence stems making up the IC in Appendix D suggests that the test is designed to evoke completions indicating levels of anxiety, guilt, depression, mood, differences in the SEP of certain stressors for the respondent, self-attitudes, and the quality of such psychobiological functions as appetite and sleep. The inclusion of many of the sentence stems on the IC test was based on certain assumptions related to the meaning of the concept "depression." Depression is assumed to be a motivational disorder, not, as it is often construed to be, a mood disorder. Mood refers to a happiness-unhappiness continuum; depression refers to a motivational-intensity continuum. Whereas mood and depression are often correlated, a person reading the morning paper filled with numerous accounts of war, homicide, suicide, rape, and poverty quite appropriately becomes saddened, unhappy, and moody. But, in spite of the moodiness, she or he is able to get out of bed, shower, eat breakfast, go to work, and play with the children. A depressed person, on the other hand, shows distinct symptoms and signs of inadequate or inappropriate motivation, such as anergia, inadequate personal hygiene, lack of interest in family, friends, and job, obsessive suicidal thoughts, and a persistent sense of helplessness and hopelessness. Moreover, true clinical depression almost always includes indicators of systemic biological dysfunction, such as insomnia, constipation, gastritis, loss of appetite, and reduced sexual motivation.

The DPSS rating scale, also contained in Appendix D, is applied to each of the thirty-five "completed" stems independently by two or more specialists in the area of depression. The numerical ratings assigned by each scorer to each completed sentence can then be used to estimate the interrater consistency for the sample of respondents of concern. However, as used by the submarine service in the past, the thirty-five completed stems for each respondent were simply scanned by the psychologist searching for salient completions suggesting depressive and other psychopathological trends. This approach to analyzing test data is called "face validation," referring to a process by which the validity of an experimental test item is based upon the judgments that responses to the certain items "appeared" to be valid for the purpose for which the test was constructed. Examples of sentence completions by candidates for the submarine service, candidates who were accepted but subsequently developed signs of depression are: to item 5 "The future . . . is bleak"; to item 12, "Things looked hopeless . . . most of the time"; to item 18, "My sleep . . . is restless and disturbed"; and to item 27, "Life . . . is meaningless."

Unfortunately, substantive data bearing on the interrater reliability of two or more judges applying the rating scale in Appendix D to each of the thirty-five sentence completions do not exist at this time. However, once these kinds of data are collected and analyzed, the unreliable (and hence probably invalid) stems can be identified and removed from the test. The DPSS score obtained from summing the ratings for the remaining items can then be checked for reliability and validity for the purpose of identifying persons with significant depressive trends and, hypothetically at least, those with inadequate SCC.

SFT (Submariner Frustration Test)

It may be recalled in the discussion of emotions in Chapter 3 (*see* also Figures 2.1 and 3.1) that negative emotions, the major component of POSR, occur when goal-directed behavior is blocked or impeded by environmental barriers (stressors). Frustration, a subjective component of negative emotions, characteristically occurs as a result of or concomitant with this blockage. One of the oldest, partially validated, principles of American psychology is the so-called Frustration Aggression Hypothesis[31]. Simply stated, this hypothesis is, "Frustration typically leads to, or results in, aggression." Originally called the "Navy PF test" (PF for picture frustration), the SFT in Appendix E uses cartoons to place the respondent symbolically in one of two interpersonal situations: in the position of the *frustrator* or in the position of the person being *frustrated*. The SFT makes the assumption that individual differences in the direction of the aggression inferred from the responses to the SFT cartoons are correlated with SCC.

The scoring system for the SFT is similar to that used in scoring the Rosenzweig Picture Frustration test, also a cartoon test but constructed mainly for civilian use[95]. Experts in the psychology of emotions classify the responses in the cartoon boxes according to one of three categories: *Extropunitive (Ext)*, aggression directed outward on the environment; *Intropunitive (Int)*, aggression directed inward upon the cartoon figure with whom the respondent has presumably identified; and *Impunitive (Imp)*, aggression that is essentially neutral, that is, has no apparent directionality.

The instructions for the respondent to the SFT are: "Look at the interpersonal situation symbolized in each cartoon and simply write in the open box the first response that comes to mind."

Examples of the use of this scoring system applied to the two cartoons taken from the twenty contained in the SFT and presented in Appendix E follow: the upper cartoon depicts a submariner in the "chow" line assuming the role of the frustrator while the navy cook assumes the role of the frustrated person. Typical extrapunitive responses to the frustrator's comment questioning the cook's competency would be, "You're damn right; it's as good as you can get at the Waldorf," or "it's a lot better than you could cook; I bet you can't even boil water without burning it," whereas an intropunitive response to the same cartoon might be, "I guess you are right; I really am a lousy cook." Finally, an example of an impunitive response to that cartoon would be, "What difference does it make anyway? We eat to live, not live to eat."

The lower cartoon in Appendix E places the SFT respondent in the role of the frustrator. An example of a typical "Ext" response to the cartoon might be, "Look sailor, this is a free country; I'll fool around with her if I want to." On the other hand, an "Int" response would be, "I guess you're right; she's your girl friend; I should have known better." An example of an "Imp" response would be, "Oh! I didn't know she was your girl friend."

Although there are a number of studies involving similar picture frustration tests developed for use by civilians, there are no known studies involving tests of this kind developed for use by military personnel. However, there were sufficient data collected from the administration of the SFT to submariners to suggest the following hypotheses: (1) using the scoring system described above, qualified experts demonstrate high agreement in their classification of submariners' responses to most of the twenty cartoons; (2) submariners with very high "Ext" scores (aggression directed outward) tend to be perceived as having a "chip" on their shoulders, a trait pattern often considered as typifying the aggressive psychopath. Moreover, this high-Ext scorer becomes extremely disliked during long submarine missions; and (3) submariners who receive high "Int" scores (aggression directed inward) tend to become social isolates, many of whom show depressive tendencies during protracted submerged patrols.

In short, semistructured projective tests using the cartoon response technique and a scoring system similar to that used by the SFT yield scores that, in a submariner population at least, appear to have usefully high validity for predicting individual differences in SCC.

STAST (Submariner Tell-a-Story Test)

Samuel Johnson is said to have once stated, "Speak, that I may know thee." More than fifty years ago, Dr. Henry Murray of Harvard University expanded this theme by making the likely assumption that important patterns of personality traits may be inferred from the content, diction, grammar, and syntax of a person's spoken or written language. Based on this premise, the semistructured projection test, the TAT (Thematic Apperception Test), was born[88]. The term "semistructured" is used advisedly to describe the TAT, since the inferences regarding trait patterning originate from a respondent's stories about the content of a series of TAT pictures containing somewhat vague but emotion-arousing themes. The stories evoked by the original TAT pictures were scored by experts according to the degree to which they reflected the "need strength" and "environmental press," dimensions central to Murray's Needs Press theory of personality[88].

Originally labeled the U.S. Navy TAT test, the nine STAST pictures, most of which involved men in navy uniform and placed singly on each page of the STAST booklet, made up the version of the TAT used at one time as part of the psychiatric screening test battery for nuclear submariner candidates. Appendix F contains the pictures (cards) from the STAST, placed on a single page for convenience.

The STAST used essentially the same instructions for the respondents that were used in the original TAT, although the TAT was administered individually, whereas the STAST was administered in groups of twenty to thirty respondents. The instructions given to the submariner candidates were as follows:

> This is a test of your imagination. You will find a picture at the top of each page in this booklet. Your task is to make up a story containing your impression as to what is going

on in the scene presented in the picture. Tell in writing what the characters are thinking and feeling, keeping in mind the following: (1) what has led up to this incident, (2) what is happening now, and (3) what will be the outcome?[37]

The STAST pictures in Appendix F were each selected according to the assumption that each picture would evoke stories yielding clues regarding the presence of selected traits or attitudes related to SCC. For example, stories written about cards I and VI should suggest the degree to which the sight of blood, injury, or even death would cause excessive distress for the respondent. Other themes hypothesized to be contained in the stories evoked by other STAST pictures are: cards III and IV—attitudes toward parents or other authoritarian figures, cards V and VII—suicidal and paranoid ideation, card VIII—interpersonal attitudes between enlisted men and officers, and card IX—degree of identification with the heterosexual role.

The scoring system for the STAST used by the psychologists conducting the submariner screening program in the 1960's and 1970's was simply to scan the stories for the presence or absence of the specific traits or attitudes assumed to be disqualifying for submarine duty. For example, somewhat detailed diagnostic interviews were conducted with the 10–15 percent of the enlisted candidates whose stories contained the following statements: to cards IV and/or VII, "This sailor has had enough of this nonsense—having to take orders from people that are borderline stupid; this time he is going to do something about it," to card VIII, "Officers always think they can cut in on an enlisted man's date," or to card IX, "This woman, like most women, constantly nags the old man." Based upon clinical impressions as to the underlying traits or attitudes suggested by statements such as these, the submarine psychologist integrated this information with the results of additional clinical test and interview data before making the accept/reject decision about a given submariner candidate.

Data related to the validity of the STAST used in this context are sparse and incomplete. One study, however, suggested the following relationships[37]: (1) candidates whose stories contained multiple themes tended to earn higher grades in submarine school than those whose stories reflected only one theme per picture. This relationship persisted even after controlling for differences in ability; and (2) candidates who wrote a story containing a suicide theme to card VI tended to obtain lower grades in submarine school, a finding that may suggest depressive trends in some cases.

In sum, the validation data for the STAST, although suggestive, is quite inadequate. Alternative scoring methods to a system that obtains scores based entirely on the frequency of occurrence of selected themes would likely prove to be more meaningful. For example, one unpublished study showed a significant positive correlation between the average verb/adjective ratio in the stories with grades in submarine school[37]. It would appear, therefore, that the diction and syntax in a story in addition to its content may be related to the performance and possibly to the overall SCC of nuclear submariners.

SST (Submariner Stereotype Test)

One study, published in the 1950's, focused directly on the problem of delineating the role-related traits defining the so-called "submariner stereotype," if indeed such a stereotype actually existed[27]. The findings from this study suggested two interrelated hypotheses underpinning the development of the SST, namely (1) the more intense and the more discernible the self-perceived masculine traits of the submariner recruit, the more effective a submariner he will become, and (2) the potentially effective submariner's responses on the SST must clearly differentiate between the male stereotype and the female stereotype in terms of the role behaviors assumed to be associated with each gender.

Thus emerged the SST, which was originally called the "Navy M-R Test," M-R referring to masculine role. Like the Submariner Frustration Test discussed above, the SST (Appendix G) also used the cartoon technique, in this case to obtain a quantifiable measure of individual differences in the intensity of the self-perceived masculine traits defining the male (submariner) stereotype. Underlying this method of obtaining information pertaining to the candidate's stereotype of a submariner was the assumption that the clarity of this stereotype was positively correlated with submariner effectiveness, including SCC.

Two of the eight cartoons from the SST booklet are contained in Appendix G. The instructions for taking the SST were: "In each of the cartoons presented in this booklet, a sailor and another person are seen talking to each other. One person is making a statement to the other. Your task is to imagine what the other person in the situation would say, then write this statement in the empty box contained in each cartoon. There is no time limit; however, it is suggested that you write down the first thing that comes to mind."

The SST was only experimentally included in the submariner selection battery for a short time during the 1952–60 time frame. The scoring system used at that time consisted of two psychologists independently rating each response on a five-point scale, presumably indicating the degree of identification with the male stereotype. For example, a rating of "5" indicated *very strong* (identification), "4" *strong*, "3" *moderate*, "2" *slight*, and "1" *none*. Each candidate's score on the SST was the sum of the averages of two (or more) independent raters' judgments of the respondent's response to each cartoon. Thus, a maximum score for the SST consisting of eight cartoons would be 40.

Examples of the kinds of responses that typically received "very strong" to "none" ratings (5 to 1 in the same order) on the two SST cartoons in Appendix G are: top cartoon, a "5" rating would be assigned to "you bet I do; you can't grow one, can you?" whereas a "1" rating to the same cartoon might be, "this cookie duster is just for show; it doesn't mean anything." For the bottom cartoon, a rating of "5" might be assigned to the response, "no way, honey; let's get this straight, only I, and I do mean *only I*, will be the breadwinner in this family," whereas, a rating of "1" would be assigned to a response such as "that's a great idea; you pull your half of the load, and I'll pull my half."

As with many of the experimental tests designed to measure the SCC of submariner candidates, the SST was never properly validated in the true psychometric sense. However, the hypothesis that the SST score calculated somewhat as it was at that time would be systematically related to the SCC of submariners still seems plausible. That is to say the face validity of the SST seems quite high. As suggested in the introductory remarks pertaining to the origin of the SST, in submariners at least, it appears that the stronger the attitudes supporting the self-perceived role enacted in a specific environment, the greater will be his capacity to adapt adequately to other environments, especially high-IED environments. In the language of ABC, the submariner will have adequate SCC. Further, it seems very likely that the same relationship exists for a wide range of civilian populations as well.

SMRT (Submariner Mirth Response Test)

There is some evidence in the older literature that the personality trait described as "sense of humor" may be associated with SCC[48]. The personality trait "sense of humor" has been variously defined as the capacity to behave in a humorous manner, to clown, to make jokes, and to have the propensity to perceive serious situations, that is, environmental circumstances containing many high-SEP stressors, with a humorous attitude. For example, the late Norman Cousins claimed to have prevented his demise from a terminal neuromuscular disease by listening for days to recordings of the "fat lady" cackling on the stage in front of the house of laughter on a carnival midway. Peter Ustinov once said, "Comedy is simply a funny way of being serious." Along similar lines, German psychologists have used the term *"ernstspiel,"* or serious play, to describe humor-producing, playful social interactions as indicators of psychological health. Finally, no less a theorist than Sigmund Freud spoke and wrote extensively about the function of humor as a very important anxiety defense mechanism. In this context, Freud and other theorists have pointed out the commonly observed fact that humorous jokes are often provoked by, or are aimed at, subjects and situations that tend to produce unpleasant affect (−AC), for instance, sex, politics, and religion. Somehow, humorous behavior seems to function as a counteractive agent for the possibly debilitative effects of intense POSR, or, stated differently, persons whose adaptive life-styles include the use of humor, properly timed, in their day-to-day life situations may have greater SCC than those who lack this trait.

A study of the personality trait patterns of successful submariners conducted in the early 1950's suggested that the use of humor by certain crewmembers tended to enhance the morale of the crew as a whole, particularly during extended submerged missions, such as the eighty-four-day circumnavigation of the world by the nuclear submarine *Triton*[136]. The content of the humor observed or displayed as the global mission progressed provided clues as to the prevailing attitudes of the 180-man crew at a given time. For example, about three days

Figure 7.2
Submarine Crewmember's Cartoon

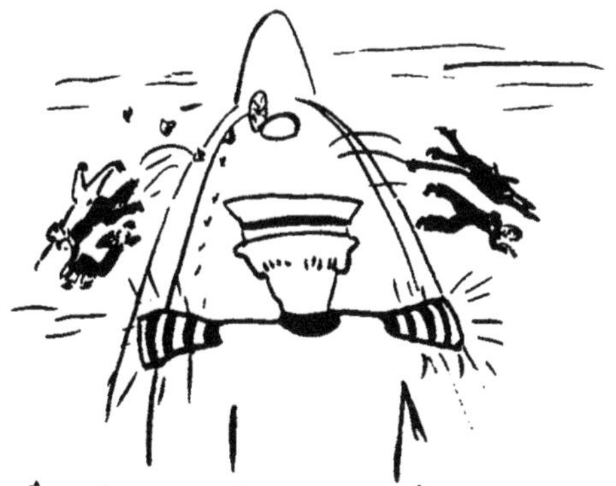
"I have good news, men! They want us
to go around again!!"

before surfacing to end the mission, a cartoon produced by one of the crewmembers was found by the author on the mess compartment bulletin board. A photograph of this cartoon is reproduced in Figure 7.2.

It seems plausible, indeed likely, to assume from this sketchy cartoon that the prevailing attitudes of the crew at that time were underpinned by strong avoidance motivation involving anticipated negatively valent outcomes ("C" in ABC), to use ABC terminology.

Additional data obtained during the *Triton* mission and from other studies of nuclear submariners (reference 140, for instance), served to corroborate one obvious quality of most humor, namely, that this type of behavior is *social* in nature. For instance, professional comedians, such as Bob Hope and Henny Youngman, have stated that they are unable to ascertain how funny a joke is (about the president of the United States, for example) while rehearsing it alone. Only when the joke is told in front of, or in the presence of others, will their social response determine whether or not the joke is a "bomb." That is, telling jokes to oneself does not usually produce real humor; however, on occasion, recalling a past humorous event in private may evoke a belly laugh. In general, however, spontaneous unrehearsed humor is unquestionably the most effective, but, because humor is a social phenomenon, its effectiveness can only be judged in social situations.

Based upon the assumption that individual differences in humor appreciation of submariner recruits correlated with the SCC of fully trained submariners, the SMRT (Submariner Mirth Response Test) was developed in the middle 1950's. The SMRT consisted of a booklet containing forty-five *New Yorker*–type cartoons to which the candidates for the submarine service responded by indicating the degree to which they liked or preferred each cartoon. Their likability judgments were indicated by selecting a number on a ten-point, vertical scale anchored by five statements ranging from "disliked extremely" through "no more liked than disliked" to "liked extremely well." (Although there are fifty response boxes on the SMRT answer sheet in Appendix H, only forty-five were used for this version of the test.)

The instructions for the respondents were:

Most people like cartoon humor; however, they differ in terms of the content of the cartoons that seems most humorous to them. Your booklet contains 45 cartoons. We are asking you to look at each cartoon and indicate on the 10-point scale the degree to which you like or prefer each one. Notice that the anchor statements such as "disliked extremely" at the bottom of the scale and "liked extremely well" at the top of the scale are located between scale numbers which increase from "0" at the bottom to "9" at the top of the scale. The higher the number the more you *like* the cartoon. Your task is to select ONE number (no decimals or fractions, please) to indicate how well you like each cartoon, then write that number in the box on the answer sheet corresponding to the number of the cartoon. Take your time. Enjoy the cartoons. There is no time limit.

The forty-five cartoons included in the experimental SMRT had been sorted independently by three psychologists into three categories according to the prevailing theme of each cartoon. Thus, the three categories of fifteen cartoons each became the *sex*, *dependency*, and *aggression* subtests of the SMRT. Because of the copyright laws, examples of the cartoons themselves are not included in Appendix H; however, brief descriptions of one cartoon from each of the three subtests follow. An example of the fifteen cartoons in the *aggression* subtest of the SMRT is a scene showing a grumpy-looking, elderly man (presumably the henpecked husband) fast asleep in a hammock. An angry, vengeful-looking woman (the wife) is busily fastening a wire leading from a lightning rod on the house to the hammock, and the sky overhead is filled with huge bolts of lightning. A violent storm is in progress! An example of one of the fifteen cartoons in the *dependency* subtest is a forlorn-looking unshaven man in a tattered suit, a large sign reading "MALADJUSTED" hanging on a dirty rope looped around his neck and dangling on the front side of his filthy coat. He is seated on the concrete sidewalk, his back against the face of a rough stone building. A large cup, clearly labeled "pencils for sale" is between his knees. The hole-ridden soles of his shoes face the passers-by. Finally, an example of one of the fifteen cartoons included in the *sex* subtest of the SMRT is a scene in a doctor's waiting room. A very attractive, full-bosomed female patient is sitting modestly with crossed legs, her skirt several inches below her knees. Tight, well-fitted hose peek out daringly around shapely ankles, bottoming out in flashy high-heeled shoes. Directly across from her in the waiting room is a lusty-looking, slightly balding male patient in his 50's, his hyperopia-correcting glasses propped on his forehead, thus allowing an unimpeded view of the lady's anatomy. Above the man's head is a serrated balloon containing the mental image equivalent of his perception of the woman's body parts. This image shows the woman's skirt far up above her knees, showing all of her shapely legs and thighs firmly wrapped in those tight-fitting hose. The SMRT respondent presumably is led to believe that the libidinous man, by means of psychoimagery, has partially undressed the seductive-looking woman.

The SMRT was administered on an exploratory basis to about 200 officers and enlisted recruits for the submarine service in the late 1950's. The average likability scores for the enlisted men were highest for the sex subtest of the SMRT and lowest for the aggression subtest. Conversely, the average scores for the officer sample were highest for the aggression subtest and lowest for the sex subtest of the SMRT. Whereas these findings were never published in the open literature, the explanation for the differences between the SMRT profiles of officer and enlisted candidates became a much-discussed topic among the submarines who were allowed to examine the data. In general, the enlisted men's explanation for the differences was straightforward: simply stated, officers tend to be aggressive men with low sex drive. Whereas, the officer group's interpretation of these results was never made known, the consensus of the research people who reviewed these preliminary data was that enlisted men in the "sub" service tend to be more "open" and less inhibited than the officers in this branch of the service. After all, the stereotype portrayed by the descriptive sexist statement "officer and gentleman" suggests that the members of this group are a "cut above" enlisted submariners and, therefore, do not readily admit their interest in, and probably, at times, preoccupation with such commonplace motives as those underpinned by the sex drive. Since this exploratory study was never replicated, the interpretation of these findings, if indeed they have acceptable reliability, still remains equivocal.

In another unpublished study submitted as a submarine medical officer's qualification thesis, the SMRT cartoons were projected as lantern slides to a random sample of twenty nuclear submariners prior to submergence, and again midway and at the end of a twenty-five-day submerged mission. The same likability scale as contained in Appendix H was used in this study. The only significant changes in the averages of the three SMRT subtest scores across the three measurement sessions were in the sex subtest. As compared to the pre-submerged average score on the sex subtest, both the midway and final averages increased progressively as the mission progressed. Again, this study was never replicated, but, assuming that these changes in the average sex subtest score are reliable, these results were interpreted by the submarine medical officer conducting the research as manifestations of the increasingly repressed sex drive of submarine crewmembers during extended submerged patrols.

The SMRT scores obtained from one enlisted class in basic submarine school ($N = 180$) showed that none of the three SMRT subtests correlated significantly with performance in "sub" school as measured by final class rank. However, the aggressive subtest of the SMRT correlated negatively with performance ratings by section chief petty officers during one submerged mission of forty days' duration. This correlation coefficient was -0.350, $P = 5\%$ ($N=30$). This finding, if sustained upon cross-validation, might be considered supportive of the widely held view by submarine captains that submariners with "chips on their shoulders" (labeled aggressive personalities by submarine psychologists) are prone to cause intercrewmember disruption during long-duration submerged patrols. Indeed, there are some empirical data suggesting that submariners with strong aggressive traits, outwardly expressed, are undesirable as crewmembers during these long submerged cruises[149].

In summary, although substantive evidence from the submarine literature is quite sparse, nonetheless, individual differences in the trait "sense of humor" appear to be positively correlated with SCC. Approaches to the measurement of this personality trait along the lines of the SMRT involving preference or likability ratings of humorous cartoons with distinct themes appear to have very real possibilities for this purpose.

SAQ (Submariner Attitude Questionnaire)

Having the qualities of motivational vectors, attitudes are inferred from predispositions to either approach (positive attitudes) or avoid (negative attitudes) the objects of the attitude, those objects being environmental situations, persons, concepts, ideas, doctrines, or principles. This tendency for attitudes to become polarized is inferred from behavior related to the particular persons or environmental situations that are avoided or approached or from bipolar responses to attitude questionnaires with response formats, such as agree/disagree, like/dislike, prefer/do not prefer, favorable/unfavorable, or valued/valueless, as applied to the objects of the attitude.

A modern outer-space-age example of the use of the term "attitude" comes from the command-and-control center's (CC) description of the in-flight trajectory of a rocket or an STS (Space Transportation System), the *Columbia*, for instance: "the vehicle has assumed the correct *attitude* or, it is maneuvering into an orbital *attitude*, or, the STS calculates its *attitude* using the Johnson Space Center as a reference point." Also, since the advent of the inner-space age of the nuclear submarine, from the CC might come the order to "make the *attitude* 20 degrees down bubble, or to make the attitude 10 degrees up bubble" or, when active sonar is being used for navigation, "make the search *attitude* 30 degrees port and starboard." Thus, there are two connotations of the word attitude, both of which are consistent with the ABC model (Figure 3.1): First, attitudes have a directional component that may be symbolized by vectors, and second, attitudes are aimed at, or are relative to, some reference point or object of the attitude.

Though related, opinions and attitudes have important differences. Opinions, presumably possessed by almost anyone in regard to something, may be defined as cold, emotionless verbal expressions of underlying attitudes[58]. Attitudes, on the other hand, have strong, often intense emotional underpinnings. Attitudes have been described as being based on "hot" motives, and opinions on "cold" motives. Consider for example, the emotional heat that is typically generated when discussing such topics as sex, AIDS, abortion, religion, or politics as compared to the discussion surrounding such topics as fishing, the weather, the acid-base balance of garden soil, or the best color to paint your house.

The bipolar nature of attitudes poses a unique problem for the psychometric design of the items used to construct attitude scales or questionnaires. For instance, most items for questionnaires or inventories are designed in such a way as to obtain a symmetrical, preferably a normal or bell-shaped, distribution of responses to each item. In contrast, items for attitude scales are constructed so as to produce bimodal item response distributions with clusters of responses on each end of the array of responses to each item. This item bimodality results from the bipolar response formats requisite for attitude scales: agree/disagree or like/dislike, and so on.

The first study of submariner attitudes was conducted by Ohio State University on diesel "subs" in 1949, prior to the launching of the first nuclear submarine, the *Nautilus* in 1954[103]. This study was based upon a variety of sociometric, interview, and attitude data, the latter obtained by means of custom-tailored attitude scales. The submariner sample consisted of 686 crewmembers from 10 diesel submarines. Of the several findings resulting from the analysis of massive amounts of data from this study, the major conclusion had to do with the relationship between the so-called "role congruency" concept and attitude changes resulting from being subjected to a high-IED environment. Briefly, the role congruency concept as it applies to submariners may be stated as follows: the more congruent a submariner's perceived role is with the expected role ascribed to him by the ship's organizational structure, the higher his individual motivation as well as the morale of the crew as a whole will be. Conceivably, it is not too great an extrapolation from this relationship to hypothesize that the greater the congruence of the three types of roles (expected, enacted, and perceived) of a person in a group setting, the less his or her attitudes will change in a maladaptive direction upon exposure to an array of high-SEP stressors, or, stated in the language of ABC, the greater the attitudinal congruence described above, the less intense the POSR resulting from this exposure to a high-IED environment will be, and, over the long term, the more adequate the person's SCC will be.

A long-term attitudinal study was initiated in 1960 to test this and other hypotheses related to the relationship between attitudes and POSR. This study involved the collection of attitude data from both crews, the blue and gold, of the *Patrick Henry*, the first nuclear submarine armed with nuclear-warhead polaris missiles[149]. The attitude data were collected by means of the SAQ. The SAQ was constructed in a series of phases. The first phase consisted of composing eighty-nine trial items designed to measure attitudes toward the navy as a whole, the crowded conditions, quality of the food, the contaminated atmosphere, and so on. Examples of some of the fifty items that remained after several item analyses are: "The submarine atmosphere is dangerous to my health, I acquire status by being a member of the 'sub' crew, I would advise a friend to become a 'nuke' submariner, the crowded conditions bother me,'' and so on. The second phase in the construction of the SAQ involved the administration of the trial test twice to the same sample of recruits in order to obtain an estimate of the test-retest reliability of the instrument. This estimate turned out to be 0.82, N = 100.

The response format consisted of a bipolar, nine-point vertical scale extending from −4 to +4 through "0" at the middle of the scale. There are seven anchor statements placed between each pair of scale numbers (*see* Appendix I). For instance, the lowest "anchor," "disagree strongly," is between −4 and −3 to "disagree considerably" between −3 and −2 through "0" between −1 and +1 on up to the highest scale category of agreement, "agree strongly," which is between +3 and +4.

The instructions for the respondents were similar to those used for the multi-category response scales for the PIB and SMRT (Appendixes A and H in that order). These instructions were:

> Please read each of the 50 statements in your booklet one at a time starting with number one. For each item or statement, decide the degree to which you agree or disagree with the meaning of the statement. To indicate your degree of disagreement or agreement, select one scale number from −4 to +4 (no decimals or fractions please) and write that number with its proper sign (− or +) in the box with the number corresponding to the item number. Work at your own speed. There is no time limit.

The SAQ was administered to both the blue and gold crews (N = 101 each) in a cross-over, control group experimental design. That is, both crews were first administered the SAQ before submerging, thus providing the control data. Then the blue crew submerged to begin a fifty-five-day patrol during which, on the thirtieth day submerged, the SAQ was again given to the blue crew. The final administration of the SAQ to the blue crew occurred just after surfacing at the end of the mission. The SAQ was also given to the control group, the gold crew, at the same time intervals, but while remaining on the surface. The cross-over came just before the start of the next fifty-five-day patrol of the *Patrick Henry*, at which time the gold crew became the experimental, submerged group while the blue crew became the shore-based control group. The same test administration schedule was followed during the second experiment.

T-tests between the mean SAQ scores were calculated between groups for the same measurement session and within the same group between the sessions. The results of these analyses produced the following conclusions: (1) in general, attitudes, as measured by the SAQ, tended to become significantly negative or maladaptive (P = 1%) under the high-SEP (submerged) conditions, both for the blue crew during the first experiment and the gold crew during the second experiment; and (2) the postpatrol mean SAQ scores for both crews showed clearly that during the three-month rehabilitation period following both patrols, the attitudes of both the blue and gold crews recovered; that is, they became more positive, reverting to the presubmerged levels.

The content of those attitudes that changed most in a negative or maladaptive direction during the submerged phase of the patrols was assumed to be indicative of the sort of attitudes that are most susceptible to the effects of the intense POSR resulting from exposure to high-IED environments. A quote from reference 149 itself (p. 186) addresses this matter directly:

> Looking at the content of the five SAQ items showing the greatest negative changes in the submerged crew, it is noted that three of these items had to do with attitudes related to the specific mission and two with long-range reward expectations from the navy program management. The seven attitude items that remained essentially negative had similar content. Taken together, these results suggest that the attitudes that became most negative during submergence and recovered least during the rehabilitation period exemplify the so-called ego-defensive function of certain attitudes, in this case, those having to do with the effectiveness of program incentives and with the enhancement of the prestige and status of the FBM submariner.

Also, further down in the discussion section of the same paper (p.187), quoting further, "Noteworthy also in this context is the fact that the two items most prone to reverse polarity during rehabilitation were those sometimes called situation-specific attitudes, that is, those having to do with the realities of the immediate environment, for example, possible, but unlikely, adverse effects of long exposure to the revitalized submarine atmosphere."

One final question that arose while analyzing the SAQ data may be stated as follows: since there were sizable individual differences in the attitudes that became negative as well as differences in the magnitude of the changes during the submerged phase of this study, what kinds of data are the most valid predictors of these individual differences? As a result of sorting through the background, ability, and performance data available for both crews of the *Patrick Henry*, only one kind of datum was found to have adequate validity for this purpose. Thus part of the answer to the question as posed above might be epitomized by the old aphorism "those who wear the shoe know best where it pinches." That is, the attitudes of well-practiced submariners with many days, even months and years, of undersea experience under a variety of high-IED conditions show rather small, if any, changes in attitudinal patterns during long patrols. The neophyte crewmembers, on the other hand, show a variety of significant, mostly negative, changes in attitudes under these conditions. It is as if the SEP of the numerous submarine stressors for the veteran submariners has been attenuated or removed all together.

A second study of a different set of attitudes of nuclear submarines was initiated, but never completed, during the Vietnam War. The impetus for the study was the well-documented set of facts supporting the allegation that a number of members of a militant pacifist group were infiltrating the submarine service and had plans for disrupting the seagoing operations of the FBM (Fleet Ballistic Missile) submarine fleet. In response to this evidence, the chief of naval operations ordered that a questionnaire be constructed for the expressed purpose of screening out these potential terrorists. Thus, the PAQ (Personal Attitude Questionnaire) was born.

The PAQ contained one hundred experimental attitude items. Interspersed among the fifty so-called filler items were fifty items that had been developed specifically to identify those recruits with strong militant pacifistic attitudes, defined as those persons who held a deep set of beliefs that *all* war or warlike activity should be completely avoided at *any* and *all* costs. Examples of these items are: "better red than dead," "I feel if struck we, as a country, should turn the other cheek," or "it would be an unpardonable sin to fire a missile at an enemy, even in wartime." The same response format as that used with the SAQ (Appendix I) was also used with the PAQ. Similarly, the same instructions regarding the use of the multicategory response scale were provided to the respondents being administered the PAQ.

Psychometrically useful normative data were never obtained for the PAQ, although it was administered to more than one thousand enlisted and officer recruits for the "sub" service. The PAQ, nevertheless, served a useful purpose during the latter days of the Vietnam conflict. By scanning the response patterns to several so-called critical items in the PAQ, for instance, the three items listed above, clinical psychologists were able, in many cases, to identify most of the approximately 2 percent of the incoming submariner recruits harboring these militant attitudes. Thus, at least some semblance of "face validity" was found for this experimental PAQ. Yet, the number of false negatives—those recruits with these militant attitudes who were not identified by their PAQ responses—remains unknown to this day.

To summarize, attitudes are bipolar motives and, as such, tend to take on directional properties, either negative (avoidance) or positive (approach) much as represented by the vectors depicted in the ABC model of stress (Figure 3.1). Based upon the submarine literature bearing on this topic, it appears that protracted exposure to the high-IED environment of the submarine, both diesel and nuclear "subs," results in significant changes in a negative or maladaptive direction in certain attitudes. Those attitudes that seem to be most susceptible to the high-SEP stressors found on the deeply submerged submarine are those called situation-specific stressors, that is, those related to the hazards that pose an immediate threat to survival. The amount and perhaps the kind of experience with these stressors appear to be the most reliable predictors of individual differences in the SCC of those required to adapt to these high-IED conditions.

8

Prevention and Treatment of Stress (POSR)

The often-used adage in sports and warfare "the best defense is a strong offense" has implications for the study of stress. Stated simply, the admonition is to prevent POSR from becoming either chronic at moderate intensity level or acute at high intensity level, the latter usually requiring immediate, professional treatment of some type. Generally speaking, preventive psychiatry espouses similar objectives, that is, primary or proactive prevention whereby debilitative psychopathology is prevented from occurring in the first place, or secondary or reactive prevention, which allows the stress reaction to occur and then subsequently applies the appropriate treatment procedures. The lay expression used to differentiate between proactive and reactive prevention is, "with the former you do everything possible to prevent the barn from catching fire in the first place and in the latter, you wait until the barn is on fire and then do everything possible to put out the fire." The time-worn aphorism "an ounce of prevention is worth a pound of cure" makes the same point[109].

The overall conclusion reached from these sayings and expressions is that the problem of prevention of excessive POSR and the treatment of their debilitative effects are intrinsically interrelated and, therefore, must be addressed together.

STRATEGIES FOR THE PREVENTION OF POSR

Referring to the basic Equation 4.1 emerging from the ABC model, POSR = K(IED/AR), and its corollary, Equation 4.3, several approaches to the problem of the prevention of intense POSR become quite apparent. The following discussion focuses on the preventive measures suggested by these two equations.

Moderator Variables and POSR (A in Equation 4.3)

As stated in Chapter 7, many, if not most, moderator variables (K in Equation 4.1) such as age, sex, and educational achievement level, are more appropriately labeled constants than variables, in many ways similar to the proportionality constant in Hooke's metallurgical equation presented in Chapter 4. However, factual data related to moderators (general health status, for example) in one way or another must be taken into account in any long-term prevention program. This is so, as the discussion in Chapter 7 attests, because moderator variables are clearly related to individual differences in the intensity and the unique patterning of stress reactions.

Therefore, an important aspect of prevention is an assessment of the probable effects of moderators on POSR. This assessment can be accomplished by a critical examination of the scientific literature and a considered evaluation of expert opinions concerning these relationships. However, in the final analysis, the contribution of selected moderator variables to the POSR together with the most appropriate prevention strategy(ies) must be ascertained on an individual-to-individual basis. This is necessary because both the SCC of a person as well as the pattern of stressors being imposed are dynamic, changing continuously over time.

Optimization of the IED/AR Ratio (B in Equation 4.3)

Selye's concept of "eustress" (literally, good stress) makes the assumption that neither the complete absence of POSR nor the presence of excessive POSR is optimally adaptive[105]. Rather, the eustress concept implies that there is a level of POSR that is maximally adaptive for each person. However, operationally defined criteria for eustress are obscure. Statistically, eustress is defined as the proximity to the population averages of the distributions of measures of selected processes (blood pressure, for example) included in POSR. Another criterion of eustress is "arousal level" or generalized tension state, a term closely related to the concepts of drive level or motivational intensity[81]. There is considerable evidence to support the general conclusion that a moderate arousal level, neither too low nor too high, is associated with favorable adjustment and, presumably, with an optimal intensity level of POSR.

It is apparent from Equation 4.1 that both the IED/AR ratio and, as a result, the POSR build up may be lowered by reducing IED and/or maximizing AR. The ABC model (Figure 3.1) suggests that AR can be enhanced by learning new adaptive behaviors, (that is, contingencies), such as PRC's or ARC's, by means of which barriers to goal-directed activity may be overcome, avoided, or circumvented. The development of more effective study habits for a failing college student is an example of a straightforward, effective strategy for prevention of excessive POSR build up.

AR may also be increased through education pertaining to the dynamics of stress (POSR) as presented in the framework of the ABC model (Figure 3.1 and Tables 3.1, 3.2, and 3.3). The educational process should include, but not be limited to, simple principles, such as: POSR are components of negative emotions caused by blockage or anticipated blockage of goal-directed behavior by environmental impediments or blockages. Therefore, in order control the intensity level of POSR, these barriers or impediments must first be delineated and then removed, circumvented, or penetrated. To do this, RC's (Reinforcement Contingencies) must be made more efficient, or new ones developed and tested. Moreover, to be "under stress," that is, to experience some POSR, is a natural occurrence for everyone at some time. Excessive POSR are seldom symptoms of mental illness, and, in most cases, they can be controlled or alleviated. Also, many stress experts, such a psychologists and physicians, are readily available should assistance be required. One outcome of this brief learning experience is often a significant increase in the person's AR largely because of the recognition of new, more effective PRC's and ARC's for coping with the barriers (stressors) being encountered at a given time.

As stated above, POSR may be controlled or moderated also by reducing IED, the numerator of the IED/AR ratio. This approach is similar to the so-called milieu therapy frequently used by psychotherapists[109]. As the name implies, the major objective of milieu therapy is to change a person's environment in such as way that the stressors are either removed or, if they remain, are modified in some way so that they have less SEP for the person of concern. The preventive prescription may be summarized in two steps: (1) periodically, carry out a SIRO or a similar procedure in order to identify those classes of stressors with the highest SEP; (2) then, for the one or two highest SEP stressors (a cantankerous supervisor or a belligerent child, for example), conduct a self-evaluation or ask a qualified observer to assess the severity of the POSR that is occurring as a result of these stressors. Examples of the elevated POSR are such indicators as nervousness, sufficiently intense to cause maladaptation at the biological level resulting in sleep and appetite problems, hypertension and the like, or, at the social level, irritability, disruptive family relationships, and peer interaction problems in the work place. In the event that the POSR associated with the high-SEP stressors do not appear to be sufficiently severe to cause debilitative symptoms, the conclusion may be drawn that no further effort is needed to reduce the existing IED level at that time. On the other hand, if debilitative or maladjustive trends are observed, selected IVP's (intervention procedures) should be introduced. A range of IVP's and SCS's (stress coping strategies) will be addressed in the treatment section of this chapter.

Expectancy of the Outcome Ratio, $RF^{\pm}/PU^{\pm}$ (C in Equation 4.3)

As explained in the discussion of Equation 4.3, the intensity of POSR is a complex function of the expectancy (subjective probability) of the magnitude and nature of the OR, the ratio of $RF^{\pm}$ to $Pu^{\pm}$. Should the person implementing the RC have insufficient information regarding the probable outcome (that is, the expectancy approaches zero), then the OR should have little or no effect on the POSR. However, if sufficient information is available to predict reliably the OR, then there will be one of two possible relationships between POSR and OR: First, if $RF^{\pm}$, the numerator of OR, exceeds $Pu^{\pm}$, the denominator, then POSR is likely to be controlled at a low-intensity level, or second, if $Pu^{\pm}$ exceeds $RF^{\pm}$, then the intensity level of POSR should rise significantly. Stated in the language of proportions, with the expectancy level high, POSR tend to be *inversely* proportional to OR. Thus, the preventive prescription becomes: by exhortation of others, by careful selection of barrier-surmounting contingencies, or by some other focused remedial effort, maximize the expectancy that the OR, the ratio of $RF^{\pm}$ to $Pu^{\pm}$, will approach or exceed unity (that is, that reinforcement will be greater than punishment) (*see* discussion of $RF^{\pm}$ and $Pu^{\pm}$ in Chapter 3).

A practical example of the relationship between POSR and the OR is presented in the following narrative. A doctoral student was informed by his dissertation chairman that because of inappropriate data analysis, his dissertation could not be defended in its present form. In this situation, the student's POSR would likely intensify greatly, whereupon, the student reanalyzes his data in the prescribed manner, thus increasing the likelihood that his "defense" could be completed successfully. Thus, the implementation of a series of contingencies (reanalyzing his data) had served to increase the expectancy that the degree would be granted ($RF^{\pm}$), while decreasing the odds that failure to obtain the degree would occur ($Pu^{\pm}$). Consequently, the proper contingency selection and application had effected a sizable increase in the OR. Overall, the result should be a significant drop in the intensity of the POSR for the student.

It becomes obvious from the example above that controlling POSR by manipulating the expectancy that OR will be enhanced usually involves finding contingencies by which barriers to goal-directed activity may be effectively overcome or circumvented. This process is precisely the meaning of the statement "E" in Equation 4.3, "Clarity of PRC's and ARC's." As stated in the discussion of phase III of the ABC model (Chapter 3, Figure 3.1), once energy associated with an NPP, the need to earn a Ph.D. in this example, is mobilized and channeled toward the identification and implementation of appropriate PRC's and ARC's (reanalyze the data and anticipate the oral committee's questions), the intensity of POSR would be expected to drop significantly, since the probability of OR enhancement would have *ipso facto* increased.

Enhancement of the Valence of Goals (D in Equation 4.3)

Goals or satisfiers become associated with certain NPP's by means of learned RC's (Reinforcement Contingencies) of varying degrees of effectiveness (*see* text expanding the ABC model in Figure 3.1). Borrowed from chemistry, the term "valence," which may take on positive, negative, or zero polarity, refers to the relative repellent, attractiveness, or neutral characteristics of these goals or satisfiers. The valence or value of goals or satisfiers develops as a function of a person's learning which RC's are and are not effective in a given circumstance. This is true because +AC, hence "+" goal valence, becomes associated with effective RC's and −AC, hence, "−" goal valence, becomes associated with ineffective RC's (*see* discussion of the Law of Effect below).

What strategies are available to enhance the valence of goals associated with prevailing NPP's? First of all, the valences of most goals are culturally determined, for instance, accumulation of wealth, owning homes, possession of academic and professional degrees, sports achievement, rearing a family, and so on. Reinforcement theory (for example, the "Law of Effect" mentioned immediately above) is centered around the general principle that the AC (affective context) associated with the accomplishment of goals serves to modify the valence of those goals, +AC for approach contingencies and −AC for avoidance contingencies[117]. Another theory, almost as old as Thorndike's "Law of Effect," is Allport's theory of "Functional Autonomy," which states that not only the reinforced goals, but also the contingency(ies) leading to the goals or outcomes tend to take on valence properties[3]. For example, the aging, retired CEO may experience +AC and consequently RF+ solely from the act of retracing the year-after-year daily trip to the corporate office, whether or not anything worthwhile is accomplished during the office visit.

Another somewhat more idealistic example of the application of the theory of "Functional Autonomy" resulting in the enhancement of the valence of contingencies for goal attainment comes from the teaching profession. Some of the greatest teachers (John Dewey, for example) achieved their greatness from their ability to generate in their students +AC associated with the learning process itself. Accordingly, for these students, positive valence, the satisfaction, the excitement, the sheer pleasure, and even fun become associated with the lifelong learning process in and of itself.

Based upon the five elements in Equation 4.3, these examples may be summarized as follows: enhancement of both the valence of feasible goals as well as the establishment of effective contingencies for goal attainment plus strengthening the expectancy of a heightened outcome ratio all combine to reduce the intensity of POSR. In turn, this reduction in POSR has the effect of sustaining the motivation to achieve lofty educational and other goals. The same general prescription for preventing excessive POSR build up may be applied to other lifetime endeavors in other fields, such as business, sports, community activities, and, for that matter, survival.

Clarification of PRC's and ARC's (E in Equation 4.3)

The intrinsic relationship between the identification and clarification of PRC's and ARC's and the expectancy of an elevated OR was discussed above in the section on techniques for increasing OR. PRC's and ARC's are defined as learned contingencies for the attainment of goals appropriate for a given NPP. In the language of computer programming, PRC's and ARC's are feedforward processes or algorithms for the association of NPP's with correlated goals or outcomes (Figure 3.1).

Accordingly, the preventive prescription becomes clear. First, identify the stressors with the highest SEP by means of the SIRO technique or a similar stressor auditing procedure. Second, since most PRC's and ARC's are learned, every means available should be directed toward learning new and/or modifying old contingencies by means of which high-SEP stressors may be circumvented or overcome.

A poignant example of the application of this strategy for discovering new PRC's and ARC's by means of which the POSR associated with localized stressors may be controlled comes from the ominous medical problem of AIDS. AIDS, which threatens genocide for some third world countries such as some sections of North Africa, was ranked as the most serious problem facing the inhabitants of the earth in a poll taken in the mid–1980's. The deaths of Liberace, Rock Hudson, Congressman McKinney, and other notables from the HIV infection have served to further exacerbate the fear (POSR) associated with this dreaded disease. Former U.S. Surgeon General C. Everett Koop in a blunt, straightforward manner presented two negative or avoidance reinforcement contingencies (RF−) for avoiding AIDS, namely, avoid unsafe and unprotected sex and avoid dirty hypodermic needles. Dr. Koop correctly predicted that the hysteria, a component of POSR, associated with the scourge of the AIDS epidemic would be significantly reduced if the public, particularly that segment of the population most vulnerable to the disease, would strictly heed these two precautions. Stated in the language of the ABC model, the POSR stemming from the stressor pattern posed by AIDS would be significantly reduced if these two preventive prescriptions (PRC's and ARC's) were recognized and implemented by the public as effective contingencies for avoiding this lethal disease.

Preventive Strategies for the Layperson

An old Chinese proverb, loosely translated, seems to fit here: "give a starving man a fish and he will be well-fed for a day, but teach the same man *how to fish* and he will be well-fed for life." An approximate analogue in the realm of stress might be: teach a person the causes of POSR, and that person will avoid debilitating stress reactions for life. In a sense, the ABC model (Figure 3.1) is a layperson's model. In what way? It defines stress mainly as emotional reactivity (POSR) caused by environmental resistance to goal-directed behavior. Accordingly, the basic equation (Equation 4.1), POSR = (f) K (IED/AR), suggests quite simply, that the layperson should periodically conduct a stressor audit by means of SIRO or a similar procedure in order to identify and rank order the high-SEP stressors existing in the environment at a given time. Having done this, one is advised to increase the AR (the denominator of Equation 4.1) by replacing or modifying the existing goal-directed activities (PRC's and ARC's) as needed to avoid, circumvent, or in some other way overcome these high-SEP stressors. These PRC's and ARC's should result in more effective contingencies for the goals or satisfiers appropriate for the prevailing NPP's at a given time and under a given circumstance. Further, the intensity of POSR should also be lowered at the same time.

Thus, for the layperson, two preventive strategies emerge: reduce the IED by identifying the high-SEP stressors in the immediate environment and enhance the AR for these stressors. How can these dual objectives be accomplished? Fortunately, the two tasks are intrinsically interrelated. A person's AR may be enhanced by the very process of carrying out an assessment of the stressor situation at a given time. Such a procedure is the SIRO technique used by nuclear submariners and others in the past. For example, while conducting graduate-level seminars on stress with some 200 students over the past decade, the author has consistently observed a significant reduction in the intensity of POSR in many, if not most, of the students following their completion of SIRO, a partial fulfillment of the requirements for the seminar. Although well-documented data to support these personal observations are lacking, there are some oblique facts and other observations tending to support this relationship. For example, the expression "confession is good for the soul" seems to be supported by the relief that Roman Catholics often report following their one-on-one confession of their sins to their priest. Further, cathartic therapy, consisting of a detailed review of past developmental experiences, particularly those dealing with psychosexual developmental and activity, is an integral part of Freudian psychoanalytic treatment for emotional disorders. Although somewhat equivocal, the overall therapeutic effects of psychoanalytic treatment for certain kinds of neurotic conditions appear to be positive[13].

Finally, there is some rather oblique evidence from the animal literature tending to argue for the therapeutic benefits of conducting something like the SIRO procedure. Hungry rats in a T-maze learn the association of food with the lighted (versus the darkened) arm of the maze more rapidly if they are interrupted by a mild electrical shock at the choice point, the lighted versus the darkened arms of the T-maze being randomly varied to preclude position learning. The rat behavior at the choice point when the goal-directed contingency was interrupted by shock was called "VTEing" (vicarious-trial-and-error behavior). At the risk of anthropomorphization, this interruption by being shocked at the choice point may allow time for the animal to consider his options—right or left, light or dark side of the maze[87].

Although admittedly a risky analogy, it may be that pinpointing high-SEP stressors by means of SIRO results in something like VTEing in humans, causing them to consider modifying old or selecting new PRC's or ARC's to achieve high valent goals. Whereas this analogy seems to be a contradiction to the age-old adage, "He who hesitates is lost," the ABC model nonetheless tends to lend some support to the similarity. That is, barriers or impediments to goal-directed contingencies (i.e., stressors) tend to interrupt or impede the behavioral vector

(Figure 3.1), allowing time for the person to back off and consider other possible reinforcement contingencies.

Before anything like VTEing behavior occurs, however, the high-SEP stressors must be identified. This is the essential objective of the SIRO procedure. An example of this function of SIRO applied to the problem of the professional certification of a nuclear submarine psychiatrist follows:

A psychiatrist with the rank of commander in the submarine service, having twice failed the oral segment of the examination for board certification, began to develop acute psychosomatic symptoms such as headaches, gastritis, insomnia, appetite loss, and so on one month before his third and final chance to pass the "boards." Upon being consulted by the doctor regarding his situation, the author suggested that he conduct an SIRO procedure focused upon his past experiences during the examination. Stepwise, the doctor listed separately on Q-cards all recallable aspects of his past examination sessions that caused unpleasant emotions for him—fear, anxiety, lack of confidence, and embarrassment, for example (*see* Glossary for definition of Q-sort, Q-cards). Some examples of the types of stressors listed individually on Q-cards were: those stressors having to do with the content of the "exam" questions themselves such as the symptoms necessary for the differential diagnosis of neurological, psychosomatic, psychoneurotic, and psychotic disorders, those asking for the dosages of various psychotropic drugs, those dealing with the obscure phrasing that certain members of the examining board used in asking questions, those stressors associated with patient/doctor interrelationships, and finally, the strategies the examinee might recommend to optimize the outcome of an initial therapeutic session with a severe neurotic patient. The second step in the implementation of SIRO consisted of Q-sorting the cards into 5 categories rank ordered from the lowest SEP stressor (rank 5) to the highest (rank 1). Totalling forty cards, the distribution of Q-cards (stressors), ranked in this manner, was examined closely by the author and the doctor one by one for each of the five categories. In particular, the content of the stressors in categories "1" and "2," the high-SEP stressors, was examined for themes or concepts defining the stressor ranked in these two high-SEP positions. None of the two high-SEP rank positions contained stressors (Q-cards) pertaining to any aspects of the common problem for most psychiatrists, namely, that of differential diagnosis of a range of psychopathology. Instead, rank ordered positions "1" and "2" contained mainly stressors dealing with the unique, stylistic manner that specific board members used to phrase the oral questions. For example, one examiner stated the prescribed dosage of a specific psychotropic drug, and then asked the examinee to indicate the likely symptom pattern a patient being treated with this drug regimen would have probably presented during the diagnostic examination. A specific example of this examiner-stylistic problem, the basis for the high-SEP ranks, is provided by the following expanded Q-card statement by the doctor conducting the Q-sort: "a female patient, age 26, a graduate student, was prescribed 15 mg. valium q.i.d.; what symptom pattern would she most likely present?" To repeat, most of the content of the 12 Q-cards in the "1" and "2" rank positions suggested that the majority of the high-SEP stressors were related to certain committee members' stylistic manner of asking questions. This class of stressors, therefore, was considered to be a main component of the doctor's IED.

To close this lengthy case history, largely ignoring the content of the stressors in the low-SEP ranks, the doctor focused his "exam" preparation upon developing contingencies for the stressors in the high-SEP categories. Accordingly, he compiled a series of diagnostic/treatment scenarios, stated in a treatment-to-symptom sequence. He then practiced verbalizing these hypothetical situations to a fellow board certified psychiatrist. Presumably as the result of identifying the specific stressors contributing most to the POSR build up associated with the "exam" situation and then practicing contingencies aimed at overcoming these stressors, the POSR experienced by the doctor decreased remarkably during the next examination session. The psychiatrist obtained his board certification at last.

In a capsule (no pun intended), one outcome of the SIRO conducted by the doctor was to identify the major thrust of the high-SEP stressors associated with the certification procedure, and, at the same time, to suggest contingencies for coping with the barriers (stressors) to a strong motivational vector, namely, to pass the certification examination. The result was reduced POSR and goal achievement.

There are additional, rather common-sense suggestions for the layperson in regard to the prevention of maladaptive levels of POSR. While treating submariners experiencing mild to moderate POSR, the author as a first approach characteristically used a simple technique that might be called "prevention by reassurance." This technique consisted simply of a series of suggestions stated in lay language and improvised somewhat as follows: point 1, almost everyone from time to time and in a variety of situations experiences POSR, sometimes quite intense; point 2, similarly, almost everyone can, and indeed will, adapt to these symptoms in time; point 3, the symptoms of stress or POSR are very unlikely to be precursors of severe or even significant illness, either mental or physical (that is, one is not going crazy or losing one's mind when POSR occur); and, finally, point 4, many social supports are in most instances readily available close by, such as relatives, friends, religionists, psychologists, and physicians.

Life-style and Prevention of POSR

The aphorism "a healthy mind in a healthy body" seems to apply here. Writings in both the lay and professional literature in recent times repeatedly suggest that the overall quality of one's psychological adjustment is greatly enhanced by the maintenance of good physical health[6]. Stated in the language of this text, the SEP of even mild stressors, as well as the correlated POSR, are greatly increased for a sick person irrespective of the immediate environmental circumstances. The goal of "wellness maintenance" has become almost a societal compulsion and has been emphasized as much as "sickness prevention" has in the past[94, 161].

What are some prescriptions for wellness maintenance and its presumed correlate, maximum SCC? Adequate nutrition, no smoking, moderate drinking, adequate sleep, and physical conditioning are some of the subjects most often mentioned in this kind of literature. A brief discussion of each topic follows.

Nutrition. Nutritional factors in health maintenance are amply emphasized in the voluminous lay and professional publications on the subject. Low cholesterol and saturated fat intake, more fish products, less red meat, very little salt and sugar, and fresh vegetables and fruit in quantities are some of the frequently seen suggestions for optimal health maintenance. By law, cereal boxes and milk cartons must clearly state the precise amounts of A to K vitamins, minerals, fats, carbohydrates, and proteins their products contain.

Lists of specific nutrients, their sources in common foods, and their possible value for alleviation of some symptoms of intense POSR are frequently found in both professional and lay publications. Some of these published relationships are supported by sound scientific data from both animal and human experimentation. Others are based upon scattered treatment records of physicians and nutritionists. For example, vitamin B_1(thiamine) and B_{12} (cobalamine), found in cereals, organ meats, and green vegetables are reported to reduce irritability, fatigue, and, in general, to improve the functioning of the central nervous system. Vitamin B_2 (niacin), having the same sources as the other B vitamins, and fish oil are said to lower low-density lipoprotein (bad cholesterol) and to raise high-density lipoproteins (good cholesterol). Still other B vitamins, such as folic acid, inositol, and pyridoxine, found in green leafy vegetables, unprocessed wheat, and in milk are said to reduce anxiety, insomnia, fatigue, and depression. Vitamin C in citrus fruits and vitamin E in soybeans are thought to reduce POSR and anergia. Three metallic elements or minerals, calcium, iron, and magnesium, found in milk, eggs, liver, cereals, and green leafy vegetables apparently function in some way to reduce anxiety, depression, fatigue, and insomnia. Finally, some research suggests that tryptophan, an amino acid component of protein found in turkey, chicken, yogurt, beef, and bananas, seems to be related in some way to generalized, chronic tension and to insomnia[32].

Also, some recent nutritional research dealing with the same amino acid tryptophan demonstrated the complexity of the biochemical interactions between chemicals in food and the so-called neurotransmitters and other substances produced by the body. A direct quote from a recent text dealing with this subject emphasizes how these interactions are related to SCC.

> If you eat protein either alone or with a carbohydrate and your brain is rapidly using up its supply of dopamine or norepinephrine it will use tyrosine supplied by the protein to manufacture more of these two neurotransmitters. When that happens, you'll find yourself responding more quickly and with greater accuracy to mental challenges. You will be more alert, more motivated, more mentally energetic and "up." If you eat carbohydrates alone, without protein, more tryptophan will be made available to your brain, which will use it to make more serotonin. As a result, you will feel less stressed, less anxious, more focused and relaxed[32, p.22].

In addition to sufficient amounts of nutrients, we are admonished to include in our diets adequate amounts of nonnutritional substances as well, substances such as fiber and water, for example. At the same time, however, we are encouraged to avoid excessive consumption of other nonnutritional substances, such as alcohol and caffeine.

One obvious variable often overlooked in this public relations effort is the fact that individuals are idiosyncratic in terms of their metabolisms, biochemistries, and physiologies, as well as their characteristic life-styles. Also, as discussed above on the subject of general health status as a moderator variable, age, sex, educational achievement level, and socioeconomic status are involved in the problem of optimizing the relationship between nutrition and health maintenance and the part this interaction plays in the prevention of excessive POSR.

In sum, although the findings in the literature relating nutrition to stress remain somewhat equivocal (the relationship between cholesterol and coronary heart disease, for example), there is nothing in the stress literature that contraindicates the general proposition that taking all possible steps, including proper nutrition, to sustain optimal physical health will assist in controlling POSR level and, in turn, will greatly increase one's overall SCC.

Smoking. More than two decades have passed since the SG's (surgeon general's) pronouncement that there was a causal relationship between cigarette smoking and certain heart and lung diseases. Whereas the studies supporting the SG's pronouncement were all correlational in terms of research design and, as a result, only suggested, but did not prove, these reported relationships, they, nonetheless, indicated that heavy cigarette smokers as compared to nonsmokers have a higher incidence of serious heart and lung disorders. However, Dr. Koop, the former SG, and others have perhaps overextrapolated the meaning of these data publicly by stating ostensibly precise numbers to indicate the incidence of deaths *caused* by tobacco smoke directly inhaled by the smokers themselves or passively by breathing other people's smoke. Insofar as is known at this time, biogenetic predispositional causes of these so-called "cigarette-induced" deaths have not been adequately controlled in the experimental data presently in this literature. For example, have carefully designed studies involving adequate samples of identical twins, one of each pair a heavy smoker and the other a nonsmoker, been compared in terms of cardiopulmonary health during their adolescent and adult lives? The scientific community anxiously awaits the results of such a study.

Although the argument being made here may have been more appropriately addressed in Chapter 9 dealing with research methodology, it is nonetheless important at this time to develop a critical attitude when interpreting the results obtained from comparative group, correlational studies typified by the smoker data. In terms of cause and effect, the results are at best equivocal. Heavy smokers differ in many ways from nonsmokers besides the small differences in the incidence of specific diseases. For example, one brief review of the literature [155] pertaining to these differences indicates that heavy cigarette smokers consume more alcohol and coffee, they have more neurotic traits, are more extroversive, make poorer grades in college, and, if married, are more likely to become divorced. Interestingly, there seems to be no significant differences between smokers and nonsmokers in terms of tested intelligence and educational achievement levels. Accordingly, a more realistic interpretive statement summarizing the smoker literature to date would be "the kind of people who smoke cigarettes excessively are more prone to develop cardiopulmonary disease during their lifetimes than are nonsmokers, but these illnesses may or may not be caused by the combustion products of tobacco."

All of this equivocality aside, however, there is no question that the social acceptance of public smoking has depreciated remarkably in the past two decades. Undoubtedly many more smokers would have "kicked the habit" during this time had it not have been for the compelling factors that tend to perpetuate smoking behavior. For one thing, the effort expended and the tenacity required to stop smoking in and of itself produces some degree of POSR. Although not effective over the long term, smoking appears to reduce the intensity of some components of POSR for some people. Thus, a vicious circle is initiated (*see* Chapter 3). Although not in agreement with Dr. Koop that the drug nicotine found in cigarettes is a truly addictive substance, nicotine, inhaled by smoking cigarettes, most certainly causes a persistent dependency at the very least, similar perhaps to that caused by the caffeine in coffee.

In the language of ABC, removing a "coffin nail," as some call a cigarette, from a pack or stuffing a pipe, then lighting up, and finally inhaling the heavy hot, tasty smoke are linked contingencies repeatedly being reinforced positively by the sheer pleasure (+AC) of the behavioral sequence. That simply seeing the exhaled smoke is strongly reinforcing may be inferred from the fairly well-documented evidence that the recidivism rate of blind, habituated smokers is much lower than that of sighted persons trying to get "unhooked." Peer pressure to conform, particularly in adolescent and young adult groups, is yet another reinforcing factor affecting the extinction rate of smokers.

Other factors contributing to the habituating characteristics of smoking behavior should be considered. One important class of contributing factors involves the psychopharmacology of the drug nicotine itself. For instance, there is considerable evidence that the nicotine content of tobacco smoke causes increased heart rate and blood pressure and reduced peripheral circulatory volume, the latter indicated by a significant drop in skin temperature and a decrease in peripheral blood flow rate. Moreover, there is some evidence to suggest that by causing an increase in the adrenal gland secretion of epinephrine, nicotine indirectly causes an increase in blood sugar with, in turn, a reduction in appetite. Along similar lines, there is also some indication that nicotine causes an inhibition of peristaltic contractions caused by hunger, further contributing toward a reduction in appetite. These dual findings would seem to support the often-reported notion that smoking serves an appetite-appeasing function. Stated slightly differently in ABC language, nicotine may serve as a vicarious reinforcer for contingencies supported by the primary need for food.

Although the circumnavigation of the earth by the USS *Triton* antedated the

1964 Surgeon General's report on "Smoking and Health" by some four years, the question of the contribution of the noxious, if not toxic by-products of tobacco smoke to the atmosphere of the hermetically sealed submarine was then, and still is, very much in the forefront. Except in unusual circumstances, such as when venting fuel tanks inboard, during certain casualty conditions (smoke in the degaussing compartment, for example) or while hydrogen is being produced during battery charging, smoking is virtually unrestricted for the 70 percent of the crews who smoke on the submarines of the U.S. Navy. However, with the advent of nuclear "subs" in the mid–1950's resulting in the crew size increasing from 60 to 140 and the submerged duration increasing from 4 to 80 days or more, the possible risk of the exposure, actively or passively, of many young men to tobacco smoke for such long durations in an autoclave-like steel tube took on new significance for the U.S. Naval Medical Department.

In response to this concern, a controlled experiment was designed and implemented on the twin-reactor nuclear submarine *Triton* while transitting the Indian Ocean during the 84-day submerged global circumnavigation in 1960[155]. The experiment consisted of obtaining measurements of eighteen indices of cardiovascular function and twenty-two self-ratings of mood, quality of sleep, alertness, and so on. The subjects consisted of two random groups of submariners (N = 10 each), one group consisting of heavy cigarette smokers and the other of nonsmokers. The measurement data was collected daily several days before the seventy-two-hour smoking curfew was imposed, during the period when the "smoking light" was out and several days following the no-smoking period. Some of the most pertinent findings from this study were: (1) the smokers showed consistently higher mean oral temperature and pulse rate, both resting and following exercise; (2) the effects of the smoking curfew clearly demonstrated significant increase in the pulse rates of the smokers but not among the nonsmokers; (3) there was no significant difference in the mean blood pressure of the two groups; (4) the smokers, but not the nonsmokers, reported a remarkable decrease in their alertness and an increase in the severity of their symptoms of insomnia during the no-smoking period; and finally, and perhaps most importantly, (5) the mood of the smokers, and to an extent, the nonsmokers alike, irritated by the grumbling of the smokers, deteriorated during the smoking curfew to such a degree that debilitative performance decrements were observed in both the experimental and control subjects, and in a sizable number of the nonparticipating crewmembers as well.

In summary, taking all of this information pertaining to the relationship between smoking and health into consideration, and in the face of the barrage of public warnings about the risks of smoking, it would seem at least prudent to avoid including smoking as a habitual aspect of one's life-style. The result of this decision may well be an improvement in one's general lifelong health status and, as a consequence, quite possibly an enhancement of overall SCC.

Alcohol Consumption. A similar life-style decision is associated with excessive consumption of alcohol because of its adverse effects upon general health and, by extension, SCC. Since the Eighteenth Amendment, the prohibition amendment to the Constitution, was enacted in 1933 to rescind the federal prohibition law, the incidence of alcohol-related injuries and deaths from automobile accidents, crimes of violence, such as homicides, suicides, and child abuse, as well as incidence of broken homes and poverty, have all increased dramatically.

Contrary to the generally held belief that the drug alcohol is a stimulant, it is a scientifically documented fact that the psychopharmacological action of alcohol is one of a central nervous system depressant. Moreover, alcohol intake in high dosages produces the systemic toxicity called a hangover, which can be very debilitating and long lasting. In the language of the ABC model, alcohol has cerebral effects that block inhibitive motivation causing negatively valent (avoidance) goals to become less negative, or even positive. The net effect for the severely intoxicated person is that socially unacceptable PRC's, such as reckless driving, wife or child abuse, and irresponsible sexual behavior, become contingencies for goals that no longer have the inhibitive qualities for the stuporous inebriate.

If for no other reason than that responsible members of society regard alcoholic intoxication as socially unacceptable, moderation in the consumption of this drug should be an element of life-style worth adopting. This element of life-style, if adhered to throughout life, should enhance one's SCC and, at the same time, reduce the likelihood of the occurrence of acute or chronic POSR at a high-intensity level.

Sleep Habits. It has been said that almost everyone considers herself or himself an expert on the subject of sleep, since everyone spends one-third of his or her life doing it. Thus, one common-sense definition of sleep is an arousal state somewhere between unconsciousness and full wakefulness. More precisely, sleep may be considered as a space on an excitability continuum bounded by a state of complete unawareness or unconsciousness on one end through different levels of comatosity to alert vigilance and finally to hypermanic agitation. The major biological functions of sleep are tissue repair and the removal of lactic acid build up in the muscles and brain resulting from fatigue. On the other hand, the psychological function of sleep is less clear, one technical theory being that sleep is a withdrawal mechanism, a narcoleptic-like or hysterical conversionary state aimed at relieving the unpleasant affect associated with the anxiety component of POSR[49].

The most precise technique for measuring the depth of sleep is by means of EEG (electroencephalographic) tracings. Under most arousal conditions, the preponderance of slow-frequency, high-amplitude delta rhythms and the absence of the alpha waves of wakefulness in the EEG record are indicative of deep sleep. Although not as precise as the EEG indicators of the soundness of sleep, there are three additional indexes of quality of sleep. Usually measured by means of self-reports of the person whose sleep is being monitored, these indexes are: DFA (difficulty falling asleep), SCD (sleep continuity difficulty), and EMA (early morning awakening). The authors of the modern psychiatric text in which these sleep-related indexes are introduced argue that inadequate sleep habits may be one of the most important causes, concomitants, or, at the very least, symptoms of most categories of mental illness[28]. They cite as an example the EMA index as a reliable indicator of the severity of most depressive illnesses. Assuming that the relationships between these sleep indexes and mental illness have acceptable validity, then the interrelationship between sleep and SCC becomes immediately apparent.

There are several studies of sleep deprivation, all of which report findings tending to support the general proposition that most people can tolerate a period of sleeplessness for up to forty hours without serious physical or mental degradation. The same literature, however, concurs that deprivation of one hundred hours or more can result in significant POSR, frequently with distinct symptoms of severe mental disturbance, such as irritability, impulsiveness, and reduced decision-making capacity. In extreme cases, symptoms of paranoid schizophrenia have been reported following deprivation of one hundred hours or more duration, symptoms such as auditory and visual hallucinations, delusions, hostility, and suspiciousness[49]. Although individual differences in the amount and quality of sleep required for the maintenance of optimal health vary from 5 1/2 to 9 1/2 hours, the average seems to be about 7 1/2 hours.

Insomnia and hyposomnia among the crewmembers of both diesel and nuclear submarines have always been serious problems. For instance, it is a fairly common occurrence for a submariner to wander around the submerged "inner space" of the "sub" without closing his eyes to sleep for many days on end[138]. The difficulty in a submariner's being able to obtain sufficient quantity and quality of sleep during prolonged submerged missions is related to a number of high-SEP stressors unique to the submarine environment. For example, one class of high-SEP stressors is noise, which, in certain watertight compartments, frequently reaches intensity levels of eighty-five decibels or more at mixed frequencies. Also, the inevitable chatter of shipmates going on and coming off their duty cycles should be added to this list of sleep-preventing stressors. In his research in the late 1940's, a pioneer in the field of sleep research, Dr. Nataniel Kleitman of the University of Chicago, identified another class of stressors adversely affecting the adequacy of the sleep of diesel submariners. These stressors resulted from what came to be called the phenomenon of diurnal flattening or the desynchronization of the diurnal-nocturnal (day-night) cues[138]. Nuclear submarines, the submerged duration of which may be two months or more (it has been said facetiously that the "nukes" need only surface every four years for the crew to re-enlist), maintain the illumination levels constant from compartment to compartment. Accordingly, in order to sustain the watch-standers' eyes in a dark-adapted condition for periscope viewing, the illumination level in the control center is almost always held at a low or "rig for red" condition. Moreover, the commanding officer of the submarine generally adopts a four on eight off, or a six on twelve off, or occasionally, a six on six off work-rest cycle around the twenty-four-hour clock. All of these duty schedules require that the sleeping compartment be kept at a low-illumination level as well as at a low-noise level. On the other hand, the eating and recreation areas are maintained at a constant daylight level of illumination. Insofar as the sleeping habits of the crewmembers are concerned, part of the problem seems to be environmental constancy or stimulus invariance, whereby the circadian (about a twenty-four-hour day) cycles of psychophysiological functions are interrupted by the removal of day-night cues. As a result, the cycles of blood pressure, heart rate, body temperature, and some endocrinological production rates (catecholamines, for example), which are synchronized to the day-night, twenty-four-hour cues while on shore, become desynchronized when submerged. This desynchronization of functions adversely affects the submariners' sleep habits, which, in turn, causes performance decrements in the majority of the crew. Thus, diurnal flattening becomes a high-SEP stressor particularly when the "sub" is under way, for instance at thirty knots, and particularly while transitting east and west when time zones are crossed every thirty-three hours or so.

The longest submerged mission of any submarine at that time in history was carried out by the first nuclear submarine, *Nautilus*, in 1956[131]. During that record-breaking mission of eleven days' duration, data pertaining to the quality and quantity of sleep were collected from a random sample of 30 of the 115-man crew of *Nautilus*. The data were obtained by means of self-reported, confidential rating diaries completed daily by each of the participants in the study.

Generalizations from these rating data suggest the following conclusions pertaining to the sleep habits of submariners during this eleven-day submerged mission: (1) although no significant changes in the average amount of sleep occurred during the mission, about 10 percent of the sample averaged only five hours of sleep per twenty-four-hour period throughout the eleven days; (2) the DFA index, on average, increased significantly from ten minutes "time-to-fall-asleep" on the third submerged day to twenty-two minutes on the sixth day of the mission; (3) the median SCD index, as indicated by the submariner's own count of the number of times he had awakened during a regular sleeping period, remained constant at 1.5 per period, although 10 percent reported an SCD of three awakenings every sleeping period of the eleven days submerged; and (4) although the reported incidence of dreaming increased toward the end of the voyage, there were no reported changes in the pleasantness or unpleasantness of the dream content as the mission progressed.

What kinds of inferences can be drawn pertaining to the sleep habits of nonsubmariners from these rather sparse data obtained from submariners during an eleven-day mission? In the first place, the data from this eleven-day exposure to the many and varied stressors found in a submerged nuclear submarine suggest that the DFA index of the quality of sleep may be the most practical indicator of the adequacy of the sleep a person is able to get during a given sleep period, particularly when one of the major sleep-inhibiting stressors involved is "diurnal flattening." Extrapolating this finding from "subs" to a nonsubmarine setting, an approximately analogous situation might be the desynchronization of circadian functions of industrial shift workers whose work cycles periodically change back and forth between night and day shifts. Thus, changes in the sleep habits similar to those found in the *Nautilus* study might be expected to occur in these shift workers, particularly if the night/day shift rotation cycle is too short, for example, three weeks or less.

A summary statement regarding the relationship between sleep habits and SCC is similar to the statements summarizing the conclusions of the previously discussed life-style elements presumed to be related to SCC. That is, since maintenance of optimal physical and mental health is positively correlated with SCC, it follows that the adoption of a life cycle that includes appropriate sleep habits should serve to enhance one's SCC and, by extension, reduce the likelihood that debilitating POSR will occur during one's lifetime.

Physical Conditioning. The number of joggers on the streets and byroads, the ever-increasing sales of exercise equipment, and the number of conditioning salons springing up across the nation attest to the prevailing belief that exercise in some form and to some degree is an effective health maintenance strategy. Although based upon somewhat equivocal experimental evidence, the voluminous lay as well as scientific literature in this field suggest that regular exercise tends to improve cardiovascular and lung function. Also, moderate exercise on a regular basis may increase the efficiency of the immune system for preventing disease, may result in the production of a class of pain-suppressing neuropeptides called endorphins, and may raise the level of high-density lipoprotein (the good cholesterol) in the blood. Moreover, exercise may favorably affect mood states. Often heard from exercise enthusiasts is something like "a vigorous workout simply makes me feel good"[72, 92].

Before focusing in more detail on each of these presumed consequences of physical conditioning, definitions of some of the frequently used terms in this area would seem to be in order. First, what is meant by "aerobic" versus any other type of exercise? The word "aerobic" literally means "oxygen in," or expanded slightly, "change processes caused by the presence of oxygen." Exercise physiologists label this process or these processes "aerobic respiration." A more precise definition of aerobic exercise might be "any physical activity that significantly increases the concentration of oxygen in the alveolar air in the lungs as well as in the blood and the other cells of the body." Exercise physiologists state that the goal of aerobic exercise is to increase significantly the oxygen demand without producing an intolerable oxygen deficit. These experts in the field estimate the oxygen demand/oxygen deficit relationship by measuring the oxygen tension or the partial pressure of the oxygen in the blood. An approximate layperson's rule of thumb for determining whether a safe aerobic state has been attained during exercise may be derived from a series of simple stepwise calculations based upon heart rate and age:

Step 1—MHR(maximum recommended heart rate) is (MHR = 220 − age); units are beats/minutes, or bpm.

Step 2—Obtain RHR (resting heart rate) from palpating the wrist or neck; the median of three successive readings is advised.

Step 3—Subtract RHR from MHR to obtain the HLR (high/low range).

Step 4—Multiply HLR by 60 percent and add RHR to obtain the lower aerobic training level. Similarly, take 85 percent of HLR and add RHR to obtain the upper aerobic training level.

For example, a safe aerobic training range for a 50-year-old medically-healthy male or female would be: MHR = 220 − 50 = 170 bpm, and RHR, let us say, is found to be 70 bpm, which is about the average for this age group. Sixty percent of (170–70), the HLR, plus the RHR of 70 equals 130 bpm, the lower training level. The upper training level is calculated as 85 percent of the HLR (100) equals 85 plus the RHR of 70 to give 155 bpm. Thus, a recommended safe training range for this 50-year-old person would be approximately 130 to 155 bpm.

Another simple test for the layperson to determine whether she/he might be approaching a serious oxygen deficit while exercising is to simply count slowly aloud from one to five to see if there is sufficient breath remaining in the airways to clearly enunciate the number "five," a labial sound requiring a sizable burst of expiratory air to produce. If a clear "five" sound cannot be produced, it is likely that an oxygen deficiency is fast approaching, suggesting that the intensity of exercise should be immediately reduced, or better still, stopped altogether for the present exercise session.

Since many of the measurements used in exercise research involve terms used in clinical medicine, a distinction between two medical concepts is essential, namely, the distinction between signs and symptoms. Symptoms are subjectively reported complaints, heart burn, headache, and joint and muscle pain, for example. Signs, on the other hand, are observable, palpable indicators of an organic condition or process. Examples of "signs" often used in evaluating the effects of physical conditioning are heart sounds, heart rate, blood pressure, blood cholesterol, sugar concentration, body temperature, urinary catecholamines, and skin irritations or color changes.

What scientific information bearing on the question of the mechanisms and processes accounting for the reported beneficial effects of programmed exercise on general health status, including SCC, is presently available? Most of these processes are physiological and biochemical in nature. The assumption underlying the somewhat detailed description of each of these processes to follow is that by understanding these physical mechanisms, new, and hopefully more effective, conditioning programs can be developed and implemented.

First, there is a sizable literature pertaining to the relationship of exercise to cardiovascular efficiency. Approximately one-fifteenth of an adult's body weight is blood, roughly four to six liters in volume. The major component of blood is a liquid called plasma, which acts as the support medium for two kinds of formed cells: the erythrocytes or RBC's (red blood cells), numbering 4 to 5 million per cubic millimeter (mm^3) of blood, and the leukocytes or WBC's (white blood cells), which number 5,000 to 10,000/mm^3 of blood. Only the WBC's have nuclei, of several different forms. The major function of WBC's is to ward off invading, sometimes pathogenic, bacteria, viruses, tumor cells, and other microscopic substances. On the other hand, the major function of RBC's is the transport of oxygen (O_2) throughout the body. Approximately 21 percent of the inspired air is O_2, which, in the process of being transported to the cells of the body, combines with an iron-containing protein, hemoglobin, to form oxyhemoglobin. Oxyhemoglobin, being an unstable compound, readily gives up O_2 to the cells. On average, one hundred ml (milliliters) of blood contain about fifteen grams of hemoglobin.

The blood is circulated by the heart, a fist-size, hollow muscular organ that functions as a pump with a "pumping" cycle averaging about 1/72 of a minute, or stated differently, the pulsations felt at the wrist or neck occur just under a second apart or at a rate of about seventy-two times per minute. The amount of blood circulated by each beat of the heart is called the stroke volume, which, in adults, averages about seventy ml (milliliters) of blood per stroke. The mechanics of the heart are much like a sponge. When it is completely expanded with the heart muscles relaxed, a phase of the cycle called the diastole occurs. At the end of this phase, the so-called diastolic pressure is low, of the order of sixty to ninety mm Hg (sixty to ninety millimeters of mercury). On the other hand, when the heart compresses, the blood is squeezed out, forcing the blood into the arteries and veins. In this phase of the cycle, the pressure is high, in the range of 115 to 180 mm Hg. This phase of the heart cycle is called the systole, and the pressure at that time is called the systolic blood pressure. Whereas cardiologists are not in full agreement as to a healthy blood pressure level, depending upon age, weight, and medical history, they nonetheless often cite something of the order of 75 to 130 mm Hg for the diastolic and systolic pressure, respectively. The difference between the high and low pressures is called the pulse pressure. The pulse pressure, together with a related measure called the stroke volume (the volume of blood expelled from the heart chamber on each systole), are also important indicators of the strength and resiliency of the heart muscle.

Although not supported by substantial scientific data in all cases, some of the tentative findings pertaining to the effects of regular exercise on cardiovascular fitness are as follows: (1) there is an increase in anticoagulating substances in the blood plus an increase in plasma volume, which, when taken together, result in a "thinning" of the blood, thus reducing the likelihood of infarcts or clots acting as blockages in the circulatory system, a common example being the so-called "heart attack"; (2) following exercise, more efficient oxygenation of the blood occurs as a result of an increase in the partial pressure of oxygen in the blood and as a result of an increase in the number of circulating RBC's; (3) overall enhancement of the hemodynamic processes results from an increase in blood vessel elasticity, increases in pulse pressure and stroke volume, and more efficient venous return of the blood to the heart; (4) resting blood pressure and heart rate generally are greatly reduced for the well-conditioned person because of a general increase in cardiac output; and (5) there is some evidence that the level of high-density lipids (the so-called "good" fatty substances) increases during vigorous exercise, thus reducing the likelihood of stroke or other cardiovascular problems. In this context, a humorous admonition, several versions of which are often cited by exercise enthusiasts, is based on an expansion of the finding that exercise results in an increase in the "good" cholesterol level in the blood. Some other findings along the same lines are that moderate consumption of alcohol as well as caffeine also results in an increase in those protective lipids in the blood. Thus, the admonition, expressed facetiously, "to avoid stroke and/or other cardiovascular complications, get loaded, drink coffee to sober up, and run like hell!"

Closely related to cardiovascular adequacy is the notion of pulmonary or lung efficiency, the two concepts sometimes described together as cardiopulmonary sufficiency. Simply stated, lungs function as bellows containing mixed gases at varying partial pressures. Lungs are a muscular system functioning for the most part involuntarily but capable of being controlled at will. The rhythmic inspiratory and expiratory cycle is repeated at a rate of fourteen to twenty times per minute by an adult in a resting state. The volume of air inhaled and exhaled during quiet breathing is called the tidal volume, which averages about 500 ml for an adult male. The volume of air that can be forcibly expelled is called the expiratory reserve volume, which averages about 1,000 ml for an adult male. After forced expiration, however, a gaseous mixture still remains in the lungs. This so-called residual or minimal air volume, approximately 150 ml, remains in the respiratory passageways between breaths and is called dead space air, gas that is unavailable for respiratory exchange. The remainder of the tidal volume (350 ml) is called alveolar air. Pulmonary alveoli are air sacs in the lungs formed by terminal dilations of the small airways called bronchioles. The oxygen concentration in these alveoli, about 14 percent under normal conditions, is a very important factor related to the efficiency of the oxygen transport process in the blood. Finally, an all-inclusive measure of pulmonary efficiency is the "vital capacity" of the lungs. Vital capacity is defined as the maximum amount of air that a person can (will?) forcibly expel following maximum inspiration. The average vital capacity in healthy male adults is about 4,500 ml.

Having reviewed the functional characteristics of the cardiopulmonary system, let us examine some of the findings relating the possible long-term effects of the implementation of a regular exercise regimen upon the function of this vital system: (1) breathing rate in a resting state is reduced; (2) vital capacity and total lung volume generally are significantly increased; (3) expiratory reserve volume may be increased resulting in a reduction in residual air; and finally, (4) quite probably in part accounting for the increased oxygenation of the blood of the physically fit person is the fact that exercise seems to increase the oxygen concentration of the alveolar air from an average of 14 percent to 18 percent or more. It follows then, with the increase in the oxygen saturation of the alveoli, the partial pressure of this vital gas will increase proportionately, thus forcing more oxygen into the RBC's and, in turn, resulting in greater oxygenation of the other cells of the body as well.

As mentioned above, there is some evidence that regular exercise may result in an increase in the production of certain substances called endorphins. Molecularly similar to morphine-like compounds, one or more of the endorphins may, like morphine, have the psychopharmacological effect of an analgesic or pain suppressant. Coupled with the hyperoxygenation of the blood, the action of the endorphin compounds following exercise may account in part at least for the sequelae, the so-called "exercise high," described in a number of fitness magazines.

To summarize, for medically fit persons, an apropriately designed physical conditioning program is likely to enhance and sustain one's favorable health status. As a result, the SCC of these well-conditioned persons would be expected to be adequate for most high-IED situations.

STRATEGIES FOR THE TREATMENT OF POSR

The relative desirability of prevention rather than treatment of severe stress reactions and, in some cases, the associated sequelae of stress-related disorders have already been discussed in the introduction to this chapter. POSR sufficiently severe to result in acute medical, emotional, or behavioral symptoms must be treated expeditiously in order to avoid accumulative, and even debilitative consequences (*see* Figure 6.1). To reiterate, basic to the ABC model of stress is the assumption that the components of POSR (Tables 3.1, 3.2, and 3.3) and the possibility of long-term stress-related disorders result from blockage of goal-directed approach or avoidance contingencies by immediately perceived or anticipated environmental barriers called stressors (Figure 3.1). This statement of the fundamental assumption of the ABC model suggests three interrelated therapeutic approaches: reduce the intensity level of POSR, increase the expectancy of maximizing the OR ($RF^{\pm}/Pu^{\pm}$), and identify and clarify the most effective PRC's and ARC's (*see* Equation 4.3). It should be recalled that a number of strategies for implementing all three of these treatment approaches were presented from the preventive point of view earlier in this chapter. To be noted also in that discussion of preventive measures is the fact that these approaches, strategies, or techniques were, in most cases, of the "do-it-yourself" variety, the aim being to prevent the POSR from becoming sufficiently acute to require professional intervention. On the other hand, the decimally coded table below (Table 8.1) presents a catalogue of IVP's used for reducing the POSR that have already reached maladaptive, and possibly debilitative levels of intensity. In most instances, these IVP's are administered or at lease supervised by professionals, such as psychiatrists, psychologists, or social workers, specializing in the stress treatment area.

As presented in Table 8.1, the notion of stressor levels, individual, group, intergroup, and organizational is based on the meaning of the concept "environment-of-a-person" or, stated differently, the environment of an individual at a given time. The environment at the individual level is divided into the internal and external aspects. The internal environment is bounded by the skin. Control mechanisms for the internal environmental processes as they relate to POSR are associated with cognitive processes as well as the unique functions of the endocrine and autonomic systems (*see* outline in Figure 3.3 and Tables 3.1, 3.2, and 3.3). As seen in Table 5.1, most of the primary stressors are associated with the internal environment, for example, pain, waste elimination, and oxygen, food, and water deprivation.

Although adjunct psychotherapeutic IVP's, usually of the supportive type, are generally included[162], many therapeutic strategies for the primary stressors associated with an individual's internal environment are of the medical variety, often involving pharmacological and/or surgical IVP's.

As suggested in Figures 2.1 and 3.1, when the person begins to seek environmental contingencies for prepotent needs, that person is responding to his/her external environment with its many and varied barriers (stressors), impeding or blocking goal-directed activity. These are usually secondary stressors. Some of these barriers or stressors are impermeable, and others semipermeable, circumventable, or avoidable altogether.

Although characteristics of stressors at the individual level overlap those at the group, intergroup, and organizational levels, they are generally the easiest to identify. Because of this fact, appropriate IVP's are more readily available to overcome or avoid them. For example, with the source of internal pain stressors localized, medical, surgical, and other IVP's can be applied directly. Moreover, internal and external environmental stressors may combine for an individual under certain circumstances. Thus, the complex pattern of stressors contributing to a doctoral student's failure to pass the comprehensive examinations is an apt example of stressors at the individual level. The elevated POSR typically evoked by such a situation will likely be alleviated by rather straightforward IVP's, such as a concerted effort to identify and correct the weaknesses in the student's performance in the qualifying examination, preparatory for the more difficult, high-SEP stressor situation associated with the comprehensives.

A group may be defined as two or more persons having common goals and as having a designed-in linkage of functions[64, 89]. In general, stressors at the group level are more obscure than are these at the individual level, since they are associated with equally obscure contingencies underpinned mainly by secondary, not primary needs (Table 5.1). For example, stressors at the group level typically involve ambiguous role delineation, demands for unrealistic norm conformity, and interrole conflict. An example of interrole conflict as a stressor at this level is the case of a university professor who is expected to be an outstanding

Table 8.1
Phases in the Introduction of a Variety of IVP's (Intervention Procedures) for the Treatment of Acute Stress Reactions

---

Phase I — Application of the Stressor Identification and Rank Ordering (SIRO) Technique
Phase II — Determination of the Minimum Effective Level(s) (MEL)
Phase III — Selection of Intervention Procedures Grouped by Entry Levels[a]

1. Individual
   - 1.1 Perceptual and Attitudinal Processes
     - 1.11 Rational Emotive Therapy
     - 1.12 Reattribution Therapy
     - 1.13 Sensitivity Training (Individual)
   - 1.2 Emotional Processes
     - 1.21 Psychopharmacological Therapy
     - 1.22 Biofeedback Training
     - 1.23 Hypnotherapy, Autogenic Training, Psychoimagery
     - 1.24 Transcendental Meditation
     - 1.25 Counter Conditioning; Coverant Conditioning; Thought Stopping
     - 1.26 Systematic Desensitization
     - 1.27 Graduated Extinction
   - 1.3 Behavior
     - 1.31 Behavior Modification
     - 1.32 Contingency Management
     - 1.33 Physical Conditioning Training
     - 1.34 Time Management Training
     - 1.35 Assertive Training
     - 1.36 Transactional Analysis
2. Group
   - 2.1 Sensitivity Training (Group)
   - 2.2 Leaderless Group Discussions
   - 2.3 Role Mapping
   - 2.4 Group Goal-setting
   - 2.5 Quality Circles
   - 2.6 Power Dependency Analysis
   - 2.7 Communication Network Analysis
   - 2.8 Leadership Style/Group Structural Fit Analysis
3. Inter-Group
   - 3.1 Inter-group Conflict Resolution Procedure
   - 3.2 Inter-group Dependency Analysis
   - 3.3 Liaison Role Assessment
4. Organization
   - 4.1 Management by Objective
   - 4.2 Managerial Grid
   - 4.3 Survey Feedback
   - 4.4 Chain-of-Command Structural Analysis
   - 4.5 Force Field Analysis

---

[a]Brief descriptive statements for each of the IVP's in this table are contained in Table 8.2.

teacher and student adviser, but, at the same time, to publish significant numbers of scholarly papers and books. Additional examples of stressors at the group level are listed as B-5, 6, 7, and 12 in Table 5.1.

Stressors at the intergroup level usually result from the conflict arising from the incompatibility of the goals of two or more groups. The greater the interdependence of one group upon the other, the greater the likelihood that high-SEP intergroup stressors will occur. For example, two identical crews of 140 men each, the blue and gold crews, are assigned to shared duty on each of the 37 FBM (fleet ballistic missile) submarines of the U.S. Naval fleet. The interdependence relationship between the blue and gold crews of one FBM is described as reciprocal, since the habitability and mechanical condition of the "sub" following a sixty- to eighty-day submerged mission by the blue crew, for example, directly affect the intercrew attitudes of the replacement gold crew. The reverse of course happens in terms of attitude formation when, in three months' time, the gold crew is relieved by the blue crew and so on. Thus, sensitive navigational and sonar equipment out of calibration, nuclear radiation logs incomplete, ballast pumps nonfunctional, and incomplete or erroneous accounting of supplies may become high-SEP stressors for the replacement crew[149].

Similarly, intergroup stressors are common between production and marketing departments in industrial organizations, particularly in the fabrication industries. For instance, production deficiencies may result in insufficient products to market. Conversely, marketing deficiencies may result in production surpluses, and so on. Additional examples of intergroup stressors may be found in B–5 and 7 in Table 5.1.

Finally, organizations may be defined as combinations of individuals and groups with a built-in linkage of functions aimed at accomplishing a common goal, such as product fabrication, marketing, or public service[124]. Since most adults spend at least 60 percent or more of their waking hours in organizational settings (work place, church, school, and so on), analysis of stressors at the organizational level is considered very important for understanding the dynamics of acute and chronic POSR. Stressors at the organizational level, although somewhat overlapping those at the group and intergroup levels, involve very rigid and unrealistic performance norms, inappropriate job design, work overload and underload, unrealistic time constraints, blocked communication and feedback channels, and faulty organizational design[86]. Role ambiguity, role conflict, violation of the unity of command concept, overly broad spans of control, obscure or blocked career pathways, occupational obsolescence, and mandatory retirement are additional examples of stressors at the organizational level (*see also* B-9, 11, 13, 16, and 18 in Table 5.1)[25].

Phase I. Application of the SIRO Technique[145]

Phase I in Table 8.1, application of SIRO, has as its main objective identifying and rank ordering the major environmental stressors in terms of their SEP. It may be recalled that an example of the application of this technique was presented in the section on prevention of excessive POSR above. The major outcome of SIRO in this instance was the localization of the stressors with the lowest and highest SEP. In this case, the psychiatrist conducting the SIRO, having failed a previous board certification examination, was able to ascertain from the SIRO rankings that most of the high-SEP stressors pertained to certain of the board of examiners' unique phrasing of specific "exam" questions. Thus, the nature of selected high-SEP stressors delineated by SIRO had served to suggest a series of IVP's that, in this case history at least, consisted of systematic, supervised practice in responding effectively to questions stated in this unique manner.

Although discussed earlier, it may be well to point out again an important spinoff of SIRO, namely, that the SIRO process itself seems to have a beneficial therapeutic effect in that the POSR of the person conducting the procedure are generally reduced in intensity. This psychotherapeutic spinoff for the person conducting the SIRO is so dramatic in some instances that the processes by which this side effect occurs has been labeled SIRT (Stressor Identification and Ranking Therapy). An old psychological principle, espoused by the early Gestalt psychologists, the "need for cognitive structure" may account in part for this effect[64]. Stated simply, this principle refers to the persistent human need for an understanding of what is out there, the rocks and shoals that exist in the present as well as those that may lie ahead on the voyage of life, to wax prosaic for a moment. Thus, SIRO yields an array of high- and low-SEP stressors, a disclosure that may function as an IVP by providing an opportunity to study the dynamics of these stressors, and to develop and field test a variety of IVP's appropriate for coping with them.

Phase II. Determination of the MEL (Minimum Effective Level[s])

The MEL concept states that an IVP should not be introduced at any deeper level than is necessary to effect a significant reduction in POSR. Thus, Phase II in Table 8.1 involves the determination of the MEL for the introduction of one or more IVP's, at the individual, group, intergroup, or organizational level.

The first and perhaps the most valid indicator from which an optimal MEL may be determined is based upon an examination of the level or levels of stressors found in the highest and lowest SEP categories obtained from the SIRO data. For instance, let us suppose that most of the stressors in the high-SEP (upper 15 percent) end of the SIRO distribution were related in some way to the attitudes of coworkers toward the person implementing the SIRO. In this case, the stressors found on the Q-cards in the high-SEP ranks might have been: "not being asked to join coworkers in the lunch-time chatter, coworkers always react negatively to my opinions, my supervisor never lets me know how I am doing, and very few of my coworkers speak to me at the beginning of the workday," and so on. It is apparent that the content of these stressors suggests that negative interpersonal attitudes at the group level quite likely contributed significantly to the IED and, consequently, to the POSR for this person in this situation. Having identified the MEL at the group level, one or more of the IVP's for the group level (coded 2.1 to 2.8 in Table 8.1) would then be selected for application to the problem of POSR reduction.

On the other hand, suppose that the general content of the stressors in the same range of the SIRO distribution was something like the following: "have too much responsibility and insufficient authority, am never allowed to participate in decisions affecting my job situation, nonexistence of any communication channels between my supervisor and me, and too many time-constrained, rigid deadlines." The overlap of the content among these stressors would clearly suggest an MEL at the organizational and/or possibly the intergroup level. As before, appropriate IVP's for the organizational or intergroup level (coded 3.1 to 3.3 and 4.1 to 4.5 in Table 8.1) would then be applied.

Another example related to the problem of MEL specification might be the content of the high-SEP stressors gleaned from the SIRO provided by an ignition system installer on an automobile assembly line. Some of the high-SEP stressors might be something like: "the parts delivery department is so slow that the assembly line is stopped," or "more than 15 percent of the parts delivered to the line have the wrong parts number," and so on. The content of these high-SEP stressors suggests the existence of a conflict between the parts delivery department and the ignition installation station on the "line." From this information it appears that the MEL is at the inter-group level. Therefore, inter-group IVP's such as inter-group conflict resolution procedures should be applied (3.1 in Table 8.1). IVP's coded 3.2 and 3.3 in Table 8.1 may also be considered in this context.

Finally, a contrasting example might be the case in which the content of the high-SEP stressors on the Q-cards was predominantly subjective in nature, such as "feel inadequate in almost all situations, feel isolated in group settings, and am tense and nervous most of the time." Based upon this content of the high-SEP stressors, the obvious MEL would be the individual level. Accordingly, the IVP's would be selected from those listed at that level (coded 1.1 to 1.36 in Table 8.1). The criteria for the selection of a specific IVP from this list of IVP's will be discussed in the next section of this chapter.

Although the determination of the most effective MEL is most directly accomplished by a content analysis of the high-SEP stressors produced by SIRO, it is also important to examine the content of some of the low-SEP stressors—those, for example, in the lower 15 percent of the SIRO distribution. The analysis of the low-SEP stressors should consist of a determination of which classes of stressors are absent and which stressors, listed on the Q-cards, have been assigned low rank order scores. Suppose for example, that such stressors as lack of communication channels in the work place or the presence of unfavorable interpersonal attitudes—both suggesting a MEL at the group level—appeared in this low-SEP range. Since they are ranked so low in terms of SEP, one can conclude that they are unlikely to contribute significantly to the prevailing POSR intensity level. Therefore, they are usually disregarded.

Phase III. Selection of IVP's (Intervention Procedures)

With the MEL or MEL's tentatively identified, the first consideration in the selection of IVP's involves two interrelated judgments: first, the severity of the prevailing POSR during the time frame of interest, and second, whether the POSR appear to be acute or chronic. If the POSR are acute and debilitative, presenting such symptoms as gastric ulcers, acute anxiety, motor symptoms and the like, then immediate medical treatment of some kind is indicated. Hospitalization may be required in some cases, or more likely, the introduction of some psychopharmacological regimen aimed at alleviating or removing the symptomatology[28]. Legally prescribed only by physicians, most of the medications prescribed in the treatment of acute and chronic stress reactions can be grouped into four classes: (1) sedatives, such as a barbiturate, for acute, agitated stress reactions; (2) minor tranquilizers, such as Librium and Valium, for moderate anxiety; and major tranquilizers, for example, Trilafon, for severe anxiety and hysteria; (3) antidepressants, Elavil, for example, for moderately intense POSR with significant depressive trends; and (4) a drug such as Tofranil or some central nervous system stimulant (amphetamine) for more severe depression. Whereas the psychopharmacological mechanisms of many of the numerous so-called psychotropic or neuroleptic drugs now in use are not fully understood, in general, sedatives affect the central nervous system; tranquilizers, the neurohormonal and autonomic nervous systems; and the antidepressants as well as the stimulants affect the central and autonomic systems as well as the neurohormonal system (*see* the outline of the nervous system in Figure 3.3).

There are relatively few examples of acute stress reactions of submariners during long submerged missions. The most severe component of the POSR presented in these cases is generally intense anxiety, bordering on panic[154]. The major signs and symptoms of these reactions are heart palpitation with pulse rates sometimes exceeding 200 bpm, profuse sweating, violent tremors, and frantic verbal outbursts, such as "I am having a heart attack," or "help me, I'm dying." Although anxiety reactions occur infrequently among submariners, the screams and agitation typically accompanying these stress reactions when they do occur are so intense that the crewmembers observing the episode have unsympathetically labeled the unfortunate patient a "screamin' seaman." Generally speaking, medication of some kind is required in acute stress reactions such as described above. Typically this treatment consists of administering a sedative, such as Phenobarbital, in severe anxiety or panic attacks. In cases of moderate anxiety with minimal agitation, a tranquilizer, such as Valium, in moderately high dosages is customarily administered.

Both the sedative and high dosages of tranquilizer medication induce muscle relaxation, reduce anxiety, and generally help induce much-needed sleep. If required, an extended drug treatment regimen with nonaddictive drugs, such as Valium or similar tranquilizers, are prescribed. However, except in extreme cases, seldom are the addictive, sedative-type medications, such as Phenobarbital, prescribed over long periods of time.

An example of an acute stress reaction occurred on the seventieth day of an eighty-day submerged mission of a nuclear submarine. A machinist mate first class assigned to the midwatch (12–4 A.M.) suddenly jumped up from his assigned task of monitoring nuclear reactor pressure and temperature gauges, and, sweating profusely, trembling, pale, and very agitated, ran to the pharmacy compartment where the submarine physician is usually found. Wildly pounding a steel safe with his bare fists, he screamed, "I'm dying; I'm having a heart attack; save me." After listening to his heart action with a pulse rate of 200 bpm and after assessing other signs and symptoms for the presence of organic pathology, the submarine doctor arrived at the diagnosis of an acute anxiety reaction. He immediately administered a sedative. He further ordered strict bed rest for three days and an around-the-clock watch for any suicidal or other aggressive behavior. Following the three-day recovery period, a tranquilizer regimen was ordered for the remaining seven days of the submerged mission.

Assuming that the acute medical aspects of the POSR have been removed or controlled as needed, the possibility of a chronic stress reaction must then be addressed. The selection of IVP(s) for chronic POSR usually necessitates an assessment of the nature of the highest SEP stressors, most effectively accomplished by conducting an SIRO procedure. The objective of this selection process is to determine the relative permanency of the high-SEP stressors identified by SIRO. To do this, it becomes necessary to estimate the likelihood that these high-SEP stressors (barriers) will spontaneously remit, or can be removed, penetrated, or circumvented. Examples of chronic stressors with a predictable remission point might be the stressors imposed on a medical school student relieved by being awarded the M.D. degree, or another example would be the unique pattern of stressors imposed upon a woman during her gestation period being removed after about nine months.

The task of overcoming chronic stressors without a predictable end point, however, can be quite complicated and leads to the second requirement for the selection of IVP's. This requirement is that the IVP or IVP's should not only control the intensity of the existing POSR, but also should provide means by which continuously or intermittently intruding stressors will be prevented from causing maladaptive POSR in the future. Stated in the language of the ABC model, the IVP's selected must in some way identify effective PRC's and ARC's for coping with high-SEP stressors as they occur. One general recommendation for maintaining adequate SCC was discussed previously in the section on prevention and consisted of outlining approaches for enhancing the expectancy that the outcome ratios ($RF^{\pm}/Pu^{\pm}$) for major motivational vectors would be sustained at a high level over the long term.

From the *Triton* global circumnavigation comes an example of chronic stressors continuously imposed for most of the eighty-four-day submerged mission. About two weeks into the trip, an SIRO was conducted by a small random sample of the 180-man crew of the nuclear "sub." One class of stressors that received high-SEP rank order positions in the SIRO distribution was associated with space restriction and stimulus invariance (sameness of sights and sounds), and the monotony of circadian invariability (day-in-and-day-out) caused by the absence of day/night cues. To allay the POSR resulting from these chronic stressors, the practice of "periscope liberty" was introduced as an IVP. Periscope liberty consisted of arranging for each crewmember to take a quick peek at the outside world through the periscope preferably as the submarine approached a landfall. For example, periscope liberty was implemented while transitting around the southern tip of South America. In this instance, each crewmember's quick look yielded a view of mountainous whitecaps characteristic of Cape Horn with Tierra del Fuego on the starboard side and several small icebergs from the south pole on the port side of the *Triton* at periscope depth. Comparison of self-reported ratings of tension and anxiety before and after the introduction of this IVP clearly showed a significant drop in both of these symptoms following periscope liberty. This apparent therapeutic effect, later labeled "cognitive anchoring," was attributed to the fact that periscope liberty allows for an expansion of each crewmember's perceptual field, thus providing an opportunity to rediscover that there is still a world beyond the two-inch steel pressure hull of the submarine. This experience seems to alleviate the confined and sameness-of-things, closed-environment feeling resulting in a significant reduction in the intensity of an important component of the POSR to these stressors[136, 138].

Long exposure to both chronic and acute stressors may also result in functional abnormalities having an organic basis. The *Triton* mission provided yet another example of this component of POSR presumably caused by the space restriction stressors discussed above. It is a well-documented finding in the submarine literature that many submariners develop lateral esophoria, a cross-eyed condition observed during extended submerged missions[101]. These symptoms are thought to be the result of the close viewing distances afforded by the constricted environment of the submarine. One IVP introduced to alleviate or prevent this visual problem consisted of the placement of seascapes and landscapes with exaggerated depth cues on selected bulkheads of some nuclear submarines. Although never systematically validated as an IVP for this condition, it was presumed that viewing these pictures did indeed expand the submariners' spatial horizon by increasing depth perception and, as a consequence, allaying or possibly preventing these symptoms. As an aside, it is interesting to note that this same type of IVP was prescribed by NASA (National Aeronautics and Space

Administration) for the so-called Solipsism Syndrome, a chronic break with reality, a dream-like state, reported by some earth-orbiting astronauts and wintering-over personnel in the Antarctic region[151].

BRIEF DESCRIPTION OF A RANGE OF IVP'S

Not all of the considerable number of IVP's purported to be therapeutically effective for severe stress reactions are supported by substantial scientific research. However, a brief statement indicating the general focus of each of the IVP's listed by level in Table 8.2 will serve to demonstrate the number and variety of intervention techniques directed at one or another of the components of POSR. Table 8.2 contains these brief descriptive statements.

Table 8.2 contains brief statements meant only to indicate the general focus of a wide range of IVP's frequently used in the treatment of stress reactions. It is to be noted that for each of the IVP's contained in Table 8.2, the suggested IVP entry level and the main processes involved in the treatment procedure itself are also indicated. In the administration of most of these IVP's, professional supervision is required, at least in the initial treatment sessions. Supervision is particularly advisable when the salient POSR indicators are emotional and/or attitudinal in nature, for example, acute symptoms of anxiety, agitated depression, anger, fear, panic, or focused hostility. Several of those IVP's are listed and briefly described in Table 8.1 under the subheading "emotional processes" and the column heading "processes involved" in Table 8.2.

After one or two orientation sessions with a professional therapist, many of the IVP's presented in Table 8.2 can quite effectively become "do-it-yourself" regimens over the long term. Such an IVP was developed and partially field-tested for use with nuclear submariners in the 1960's and 1970's. This so-called MPTRP (Myoperceptual Tension Reduction Procedure) is described in the following section.

A DO-IT-YOURSELF IVP FOR POSR REDUCTION

The MPTRP is similar to the PR ("Progressive Relaxation") technique developed by Dr. E. Jacobson in 1938[57]. Both of these procedures are based upon two aspects of the differences between tense or nontense or unrelaxed and relaxed muscles: first, differences in the perception of tense and nontense muscles and, second, the differences in the electromyographic tracings produced by tense and relaxed muscle. In a tense condition, muscles produce relatively high-frequency and high-amplitude electrical impulses that are transmitted to the brain. If intense and of long duration, these impulses, in turn, contribute to unpleasant, uptight feelings. Also, after a time, these subjective feelings may contribute significantly to a reduction in a person's SCC. However, if this muscular tension is removed, the electroneural impulses to the motor area of the brain are reduced in frequency and voltage (amplitude) or, in some cases, practically dissipated

Table 8.2
IVP's (Intervention Procedures) for POSR

IVPs	LEVEL(s)	PROCESSES INVOLVED	DESCRIPTIVE STATEMENTS
1. Rational Emotive Therapy[33, 34]	Individual	Beliefs Self Verbalizations	Focus is upon the removal of irrational beliefs which cause the anxiety component of POSR.
2. Reattribution Therapy[93]	Individual	Beliefs Attitudes	Focus is upon the identification of the causal factors to which POSR may be attributed.
3. Sensitivity Training[45]	Individual	Perception, Introspection, Feedback	Focus is upon understanding the affective component of POSR as it related to intra- and interpersonal perception.
4. Psychopharmacological Therapy[28]	Individual	Psychological and Physiological Processes	Medications are administered to alleviate the neurophysiological and affective components of POSR.
5. Biofeedback Training[17, 42]	Individual	Learning Operant Conditioning	Focus is upon teaching persons to control largely involuntary components of POSR (e.g. pulse) by providing cues as to changes in that response.
6. Hypnotherapy[18]	Individual Group	Suggestion Perception	A hypnotic trance state is induced followed by the introduction of post-hypnotic suggestions that a specified symptom will have been removed upon return to a normal arousal state.
7. Autogenic Training[93, 100]	Individual	Autohypnosis Psychoimagery Conditioning	Focus is upon teaching techniques for developing somatic sensations (e.g. warmth) in extremities which, in turn, reduces the muscular tension component of POSR. Shallow hypnotic states are often induced at the same time.

Table 8.2 (continued)

IVPs	LEVEL(s)	PROCESSES INVOLVED	DESCRIPTIVE STATEMENTS
8. Psychoimagery[85]	Individual Group	Mental Imagery Conditioning Suggestion	Focus is upon learning to develop mental images of pleasant or unpleasant situations (e.g. maggots in a cocktail to produce an aversion to alcohol or winning the lottery to alleviate depression). Alcohol abuse and depression are often associated with chronic POSR.
9. Transcendental Meditation[125]	Individual Group	Psychoimagery Conditioning Suggestion	Focus is upon producing a meditative state by concentrating on a "mantra", a single word, sound, or thought thus reducing distractions and tension, often concomitants of POSR.
10. Counter-Conditioning[159, 160]	Individual	Classical or Pavlovian Conditioning	Focus is upon changing the avoidance component of POSR to approach behavior conditioned to the stressor situation.
11. Coverant Conditioning[54, 93]	Individual	Operant or Skinnerian Conditioning Psychoimagery	Focus is upon reinforcing a coverant (covert operant) by a subsequent thought or image, (e.g. a pleasant thought reinforced by another pleasant thought or blocking an unpleasant thought reinforced by a pleasant thought or image).
12. Thought Stopping[93, 97]	Individual	Aversive Conditioning	Focus is upon disrupting obsessive thinking, sometimes a part of POSR. By saying or simply thinking the word "STOP" following an obsessive thought, produces this disruption. Reinforcing the thought stopping event by a subsequent pleasurable thought or image may be an addendum in some cases.

13. Systematic Desensitization[159, 160]	Individual	Muscular Relaxation Classical Conditioning	The focus is upon the anxiety component of POSR. Deep muscular relaxation is substituted for the anxiety associated with a specific stressor.
14. Graduated Extinction[93, 102]	Individual	Operant Conditioning	The focus is upon the extinction of the stressor avoidance response reinforced by anxiety reduction. The subject gradually approaches the stressor while, at the same time, the avoidance behavior is being inhibited.
15. Behavioral Modification[160]	Individual	Classical and Operant Conditioning	A generic term including both classical and operant conditioning techniques for changing the behavioral components of POSR.
16. Contingency Management[93]	Individual Group	Operant Conditioning	The focus is upon reinforcing contingencies that enhance SCC and upon extinguishing those that do not. This behavior management approach is sometimes called "shaping" behavior.
17. Physical Conditioning[85]	Individual Group	Muscular Exercise	The focus is upon enhancing general health status by systematic muscular exercise designed to improve cardiovascular and cardiopulmonary efficiency and, at the same time, reduce the tension associated with POSR.
18. Time Management[99]	Individual Group	Task Definition and Prioritizing	The focus is upon alleviating the POSR resulting from work overload and underload stressors by identifying and prioritizing daily tasks.

Table 8.2 (continued)

IVPs	LEVEL(s)	PROCESSES INVOLVED	DESCRIPTIVE STATEMENTS
19. Assertive Training[93]	Individual	Interpersonal Communication Strategies Counter-conditioning	The focus is upon reducing the inhibitive motivation and accompanying POSR occurring in interpersonal situations by teaching socially acceptable communication techniques.
20. Transactional Analysis[14]	Individual Group	Self-perception Interpersonal Interactions	Interpersonal conflict and associated POSR are avoided by teaching which of 3 ego-states (parent, adult, child) is optimally adaptive in specified interpersonal situations.
21. Sensitivity Training[93]	Group	Interpersonal Attitudes Self-perception Social Perception Feedback	The focus is upon the dynamics of interpersonal attitudes which may be affected by POSR. The relationship between perception of self and social feedback is emphasized.
22. Leaderless Group Discussions (LGD)[9]	Group	Leadership Communication	The focus is upon the identification and alleviation of the adverse effects of POSR on group cohesion and communication networks. LGDs are carried out and the emergence of leadership behavior noted.
23. Role Mapping[11]	Group	Role Delineation Group Structure	The focus is upon role definition, the lack of which is the cause of role ambiguity and role conflict, stressors which tend to produce an increase in the intensity of POSR.
24. Group Goal Setting[74]	Group	Goal Definition Clarification of Modes-to-Goals	Focus is upon group goal definition and modes-to-goals role assignments for each group member. The SEP of role ambiguity stressors is reduced producing a decrease in POSR intensity.

25. Quality Circles[110]	Group Organization	Problem Identification and Solution	Focus is upon identification and solution of problems adversely affecting group performance, problems which may cause significant POSR for some group members.
26. Power Dependency Analysis[63]	Group Organization	Mapping of power distribution	Focus is upon identification of power sources, power distribution and power delegation within groups. Ineffective use of power may be a high-SEP stressor for some group members.
27. Communication Network Analysis[10]	Group Organization	Analysis of communication channels and feedback mechanisms Content Analysis	Focus is upon analysis of the encoding, decoding, and transmission mechanisms. Communication channels and network patterns are delineated. Obscure networks and blocked communication channels may be a source of high-SEP stressors in some organizations.
28. Leadership Style and Group Structural Fit Analysis[35, 55]	Group Organization	Job Analysis Leadership Style Analysis Organizational Structural Analysis	Focus is upon the incongruity of leadership style, job requirements, and organizational structure. Fitting appropriate leadership style to the job and organizational characteristics reduces the POSR caused by this incongruity.
29. Inter-group Conflict Resolution Procedure[116]	Inter-group Organization	Phase of Conflict: latent or manifest cause(s)	Focus is upon the nature of the groups involved, conflict intensity, and the phase of the conflict (latent/manifest). Conflict resolution techniques, collaborative to confrontational, are applied to lower the POSR.

Table 8.2 (continued)

IVPs	LEVEL(s)	PROCESSES INVOLVED	DESCRIPTIVE STATEMENTS
30. Inter-group Dependency Analysis[63]	Inter-group Organization	Group Interdependence Analysis	The focus is upon the nature of the group interdependency: pooled, sequential, or reciprocal, the latter relationship most apt to produce inter-group conflict and consequently, high intensity POSR.
31. Liaison Role Assessment[2]	Inter-group Organization	Role analysis Inter-group Communication	The focus is upon the delineation of the linking or boundary spanning roles within organizations and between organizations and the external environment. Role ambiguity, a high-SEP stressor, may be largely eliminated.
32. Management by Objective[48]	Organization	Organizational goal setting	The focus is upon identifying organizational goals and modes-to-goals aimed at improving overall organizational effectiveness thereby reducing the intensity of POSR for some members of the organization.
33. Managerial Grid[16]	Organization	Classification of Leadership Style	The focus is upon typing a person's leadership style based largely on attitude data indicating the tendency to emphasize "people" considerations versus "task performance" considerations. Relative balance between the two orientations is assumed to be related to SCC.

34. Survey Feedback[90]	Organization	Problem localization	The focus is upon localizing performance and other deficiencies in the workplace based upon questionnaire data obtained from all organizational members. The nature of these deficiencies is fedback to the members for correction. The SCC of group members is thereby enhanced.
35. Chain of Command Structural Analysis[10]	Organization	Chain of Command outline Responsibility/Authority designation Depiction of Communication channels	The focus is upon maximizing organizational effectiveness by clearly delineating the chain of command, the responsibility/authority relationships and the existing communication network. Individual and group SCC tends to be correlated with organizational effectiveness.
36. Force Field Analysis[70]	Individual Group Inter-group Organization	Analysis of positive (+) and negative (-) forces for change	The focus is upon "+" and "-" motivational vectors within the force fields (fig. 2.1, this text) at all 4 environmental levels. Balanced forces tend to be associated with high SCC; imbalanced forces with elevated POSR.

altogether. The subjective tension at the same time is reduced and, as a result, SCC is increased.

In time, however, almost everyone adapts to high muscular tension, similar to the way we adapt to the weight of our clothing supported by the body, so that eventually we do not notice the sensations originating from the surface of the body. Stated simply, few people have seldom been made aware of how a nontense muscle feels. In contrast, however, almost everyone knows how uncomfortable a tense muscle may feel.

MPTRP is a method by which a person can teach himself or herself to concentrate on these tense and nontense feelings in the muscles. The goals of this procedure are twofold: first, to provide the person with a technique for first inducing a high-tension state in a specified muscle group and, upon command, instantly remove the tense sensations, and second, by conditioning, to associate a thought or a word (similar to the "mantra" in Transcendental Meditation) as a conditioning stimulus to be coupled with an induced TRS (Tension Reduced State)[125]. MPTRP differs from the PR technique in the manner in which the instructions for producing a TRS are presented to the subject[57]. Both MPTRP and PR instruct the subject to "make a designated set of muscles *tense*," using similar jargon, for example, "make a tight fist, tighter, tighter . . . " and so on. The PR instructions following the tension induction phase, however, are quite different from those used in MPTRP. In PR, the instructions consist simply of the vague general command "relax, relax as much as you can." The vagueness or nonspecificity of the command "relax" becomes apparent when one attempts to answer the question, what, exactly, does it mean "to relax"? In contrast, the tension induction and the post-tension phases for MPTRP consist of six discrete steps as follows: (1) make a *specific muscle group* very tense; (2) feel, experience, and concentrate on the sensations originating from *that specific muscle group*; (3) suddenly (not slowly) release or get rid of this specific tension; (4) now focus on, and contrast the difference between the feeling of a tense as compared to a nontense muscle; (5) notice how pleasant and comfortable the nontense muscle group feels; and (6) take a *deep sigh* (of relief)—notice how comfortable and tension-free you have become. These six steps or phases for one muscle group are summarized in shortened form below:

1. MT—make tension phase
2. FT—focus on the feeling of a tense muscle
3. RT—*sudden* release of the tension in the muscle
4. T-NT—tense/nontense muscle comparison
5. P-NT—notice pleasantness of nontense muscle
6. DS—deep sigh (of relief)

To be noted in the six-step instructions used by MPTRP is that instead of the general command "relax," MPTRP makes the specific request to *remove*, *re-*

lease, and *eliminate* a *specific* feeling or sensation in a *localized* muscle group. As indicated above, this is a definitive request as contrasted with the obscure requirement "relax" used by PR. In fact, being asked to relax may require an additional focused, voluntary effort to act, which, in and of itself, may increase rather than decrease the muscular tension. Again, in contrast to PR, MPTRP requires the much easier task of getting rid of a localized tense feeling in a clearly specified muscle.

To be noted also in the MPTRP instructions is that step six, "take a deep sigh," has been added. For reasons not completely understood, the deep sigh, coded DS, seems to produce some sort of relief experience for most persons, an experience something like that of "the draining off of tension." The pleasant subjective feeling of relief associated with the DS may be in part related to the fact that the DS is an expulsive respiratory maneuver resulting in the release of expired air containing a high concentration of carbon dioxide, a toxic gas. Like normal breathing, the DS may be both voluntary or involuntary, both of which seem to have a tension-reducing effect under certain conditions.

MPTRP, in the early phases at least, involves the application of the six-step routine to each of four muscle groups one at a time. The recommended setting for the administration of MPTRP is a dimly lighted room with the subject seated comfortably in a soft armchair. Eyes should be kept closed as much as possible. Hands should not touch; they should rest loosely on the knees. The subject should always concentrate on the specific sensations or feelings in the specified muscles—tense during the induction phase, nontense during the release phase.

To begin MPTRP, it is suggested that the subject take three deep breaths with eyes closed, after which the introductory phase of MPTRP begins. It is to be understood that the therapist leads the subject through all of the phases of MPTRP only for two or three sessions, and a few more in some rare instances. Following these orientation sessions, almost everyone can, and usually does, continue the tension reduction sessions on his or her own.

Introductory phase. This phase of MPTRP is sometimes called the psychoimagery phase. The subject is instructed to develop a mental image of himself/herself taking a hot shower. "The hot water is refreshingly flowing through your hair, down your face and neck, your upper arms, lower arms, your hands and off the tip of your fingers, down your back and chest, abdomen, buttocks, thighs, calves, ankles, and finally, off your feet and toes. You feel the tension leaving your body with the soothing, running hot water—like water running off a duck's back. You are feeling refreshed and tension-free, very much as if you really had taken a hot shower."

With the subject relatively tension-free following the hot shower developed by psychoimagery and with eyes still closed, the next phase of MPTRP begins. It should be noted that the following format for tension reduction, muscle by muscle, although somewhat modified, is quite similar to the one found in reference number fifteen.

Tension Reduction by Muscle Groups

Group I. Arms and hands

Hands. With your eyes still comfortably closed and elbows at 45°, make a tight fist with both hands. Hold them tightly closed; pull tighter, still tighter, hold for about seven seconds (count to seven). Closely concentrate on the feeling of tension. Quickly remove the tension as completely as possible. Contrast the feeling of a nontense versus a tense muscle. Enjoy the pleasantness of the feeling of a nontense muscle. Finally, give a deep sign of relief that the tension now has been removed from these muscles. The sequence is the one described above, the six-step sequence: MT, FT, RT, T-NT, P-NT, and DS. Preferably, eyes should remain closed throughout the remainder of the tension reduction routines. With eyes closed, it is much easier to concentrate on the tense/nontense feelings in each muscle.

Biceps. Press both elbows down on the arms of the chair as hard as possible. Harder! Harder! Now hold that position (count to seven). Now quickly remove the tension from these muscles, that is, complete the sequence: MT, FT, RT, T-NT, P-NT, and DS. At this point, it might enhance the tension reduction to let your arms dangle loosely, shake them limply, make them feel heavy, very heavy, tension-free . . . heavier, heavier, heavier . . . now note if any of the tense feelings you have induced are still present in these muscles. If they still persist, it is advisable to repeat the two manipulations just completed. If, on the other hand, these muscles are tension-free, place your hands comfortably on your lap or chair arms (do not let hands touch) and proceed to the next muscle group.

Group II. Face, neck, shoulders, and chest

Face and Collar Bone. Wrinkle forehead (frown), squint eyes, and wrinkle nose. At the same time, bite teeth together and pull back the corner of your mouth as hard as possible. Finally, raise your shoulders (imagine you are a side of beef hanging from a meat hook). Now, make both the facial and collar bone muscles tight, very tight (MT phase), hold it (count to seven), FT, RT, T-NT, P-NT, and DS.

Neck and Throat. Oppose the front neck muscles in the back-of-neck muscles by pushing the chin toward the chest without touching the chest. Push harder! Harder! Hold it (count to seven), FT, RT, T-NT, P-NT, and DS.

Chest and Shoulder. Try to touch your shoulder blades together in the back. Hold them together, tighter, still tighter . . . hold it (count to seven), FT, RT, T-NT, P-NT, and DS. Now let your head and neck "bob" down, very loose—like your head is about to fall off—like you're about to nod off to sleep. Again, as before, note if any tension still remains in any of the group II muscles, and, if so, repeat the appropriate manipulations to remove the tension.

Group III. Abdomen and buttocks

Abdomen and Buttocks. Simply make your lower abdomen (stomach) hard, very hard, and, at the same time, make both buttocks hard, very hard. Hold it! (count to seven), FT, RT, T-NT, P-NT, and DS. As before, check for residual tension in the group III muscles and repeat the MPTRP manipulations as necessary.

Group IV. Thighs, calves, and feet

Thighs, Calves, and Feet. Counterpose front and back of leg muscles by lifting your leg off the chair and turning your feet inward. At the same time, forcefully point your toe end of your foot toward your head and curl your toes under your foot, trying to touch the ball of your foot with them. Pull all of these muscles tight, very tight, at the same time. Hold them (count to 7), FT, RT, T-NT, P-NT, and DS. Reapply the MPTRP sequence to any of the group IV muscles that still feel tense.

Three Final Phases of MPTRP

I. Tension Inventory Phase. Still with eyes closed, ascertain if there still remain some "tense spots" in any of the four muscle groups. If so, repeat the appropriate manipulations to remove that tension. If no significant tense areas are localized, go on to the next phase.

II. Mental Image Phase. Again, recall that mental images are easier to develop and sustain if your eyes remain closed. For a second, it is suggested that you again develop a mental image of yourself taking a hot, refreshing shower. As the hot water drains down your head, arms, chest, back, legs, and feet, visualize the tension draining off with the hot water. Hold this image for a few minutes and, if tense areas are felt, try to remove them by means of the techniques used during the muscle tension reduction phase.

Then, develop a second mental image, this time an image of the most pleasant, peaceful, and enjoyable situation you have ever experienced, such as lying on a warm beach, fishing on a calm lake, and so on—any extremely pleasant scene you have experienced. Then find a single word to describe this scene, for example, "cool, calm, tranquil, or placid," any descriptive word. This is your private word, which need not be spoken but only silently visualized. Your private word becomes a "cue word" or a conditioning stimulus, which, with time and practice, will acquire the capacity to rearouse the deep TRS which you have learned to develop. Also, try to associate your private cue word with the two mental images you just developed, the relaxing shower and the most pleasant scene. In sum, your private cue word, when visualized or spoken, will cause the TRS and the two mental images (shower and pleasant scene) to become associated. Particularly in stressful situations in the future, saying your private word vocally or subvocally (or simply "thinking" the word) will rearouse the tension-free, comfortable state that you have learned to develop for yourself. In addition, the two mental images should also reappear in your imagination. In this way, your cue word will be instrumental in significantly increasing your capacity to cope with most stressors you will encounter in the future.

III. Termination Phase. You are now ready to terminate the MPTRP, which, after some practice, can be completed in one to three minutes, while waiting in a doctor's office (closed eyes will give the appearance that you are napping), before breakfast, before going to sleep, and so on. As implied above, with experience, all of the four muscle groups can be made relatively tension-free in an instant, almost at any time, by simply thinking your cue word.

To terminate, simply count from one to five. On the count of three, move your lower extremities, on four, move your shoulders and head, and on the count of five, your eyes will automatically open. You will feel very comfortable, like you have had a refreshing nap. You will be tension-free!

The question arises, "is MPTRP valid for the purposes for which it was developed, namely, to provide a person a rather simple procedure by which possibly debilitating POSR may be controlled or prevented?" Unfortunately, substantial scientific data bearing on this question have not as yet been reported in the submarine literature. Nonetheless, some preliminary observational data are at least suggestive of the possibilities of MPTRP for POSR prevention and treatment.

After one or two practice sessions supervised by a qualified therapist, most submariners treated with MPTRP report that the six-step tension reduction procedure, muscle group by muscle group, is easily learned. Moreover, most submariners who have learned and practiced MPTRP report reduced tension and anxiety, less irritability, improved appetite, and better quality of sleep. Also, although six to eight practice sessions were required for the conditioning phase of MPTRP to become established, once learned, the association or conditioning of the acquired TRS with the private cue word as the conditioning stimulus usually becomes quite permanent. Again largely based upon anecdotal information, most submariner subjects have reported favorable signs of a reduction in the intensity level of POSR, signs such as reduction in breathing rate, blood pressure, and pulse.

In the 1970's, the MPTRP was the treatment of choice for some forty submariners who had developed rather severe phobic symptoms associated with various aspects of submarine duty. For example, one missileman assigned to an FBM "sub" developed acute phobic symptoms, such as tremor, tachycardia, nausea, and profuse sweating, following an incident involving the flooding of the missile compartment that was his duty station. Subsequent to that event, essentially the same symptom and sign pattern reappeared each time the submariner entered the missile compartment. In fact, the symptoms became so severe that he required hospitalization for an extended period.

After being treated by several types of psychotropic drugs, such as Librium and Tofranil, for some months, upon re-entering the missile compartment, the phobic symptoms continued to reappear undiminished in intensity[28]. Eventually the medical treatment was discontinued, and the missileman was referred for treatment by the MPTRP. Three orientation sessions were carried out, after which the subject was able to achieve a deep TRS by subvocally "thinking" his private cue word. At that point, the graduated extinction procedure was initiated (IVP number 14 in Table 8.2)[93]. In applying the graduated extinction procedure to this case, the following steps were taken: (1) several practice sessions resulted in the subject's being able to achieve a very deep TRS in a matter of a minute or so; (2) this TRS was associated with his cue word plus a mental image of a pleasant scene by conditioning so that, with practice, vocally or subvocally recalling his cue word did, in turn, cause the TRS and the scene to become established; (3) then a mental image of the compartment adjacent to the missile compartment on his "sub" was developed, and concentration techniques for sustaining the image repeatedly practiced; (4) with a deep TRS well established and conditioned to his cue word, another mental image of his moving closer, closer, and still closer to the missile compartment hatch was produced—again, repeated practice in sustaining this image associated with the induced TRS was carried out; and, finally (5) a mental image of the missileman entering and stepping through the hatchway into the missile compartment itself was developed and repeatedly reproduced, being sure that the cue word/TRS and pleasant image conditioned association was maintained during the practice sessions.

Thus, the triadic association of the cue word conditioning stimulus with the deep TRS with the pleasant scene image all had become coalesced with the image of the phobic-inducing missile compartment. As a result, the debilitative avoidance motivational vector, that is, the phobia, should have been weakened and possibly removed completely.

After three sessions using this graduated extinction technique, the submariner was able to enter the missile compartment free from perceptible phobic symptoms and signs. On the few occasions when mild phobic symptoms did reoccur upon entering the missile compartment, the missileman subvocally recalled his cue word, which, in most instances, resulted in a satisfactory TRS. Most important, however, seldom, if ever, did acute phobic symptoms reoccur when this technique was used. A six-month follow-up showed no reoccurrence of the phobic pathology. Moreover, the on-station performance ratings of this missileman while participating in the fire control drills held during this time frame received performance ratings averaging 3.9 (4.0 maximum), demonstrating excellent overall quality of adjustment to the submarine environment. The intensity level of the POSR had been satisfactorily controlled.

GADGETRY FOR POSR FOR THE LAYPERSON

In 1929, Hans Berger discovered that the billions of neurons in the brain produced measurable electroneural discharges[12]. Soon after, many technological advances in the field of electrophysiological instrumentation resulted in the ability to record these so-called Berger Rhythms or brain waves on a rotating drum. With the advent of computers in the 1960's and 1970's, the technology was further advanced not only to record brain waves, the so-called EEG, but also to digitize the major parameters of these neural impulses, such as amplitude, frequency, and variability[111].

The most important brain wave pattern from the standpoint of stress management is the alpha wave or alpha rhythm. Sometimes called the "normal" brain wave, alpha rhythms characteristically have low variability and a frequency in the ten to twelve CPS (cycles per second) range. Alpha occurs for a person with eyes closed and in a relaxed but awake state. Drifting off to sleep, opening one's eyes in a lighted space, or simply being asked to concentrate on a thought or to develop any kind of mental image temporarily blocks alpha waves. Of significance for submariners is the fact that alpha blocking time is increased by an elevation in the carbon dioxide tension in the blood, a finding suggesting that alpha production may be related to pulmonary sufficiency, a topic touched upon in the section on prevention. Some additional relationships between alpha wave generation and POSR will be discussed in the section on biofeedback below.

Another source of bioelectric impulses important for POSR management is muscle tissue[111, 157]. In general, muscles in a relaxed condition produce impulses with frequencies of 8 to 12 cps and voltages in the range of 375 to 450 mv (microvolts). In a tense state, on the other hand, the same muscles produce impulses with a frequency of 90 to 120 cps and at a voltage of 800 to 900 mv. The recordings of these muscle potentials are called EMG's (electromyograms), which serve as analogue data from which the tension state of specified muscle groups, such as those employed in MPTRP, may be inferred.

Additional apparatus designed to measure a number of other indexes of the intensity of selected components of POSR has been available to the layperson for some time[83]. For example, several companies have marketed sensitive instruments to measure blood pressure, heart rate, and skin temperature. Rather simple equipment, easily operable by the nonprofessional, is also procurable for the purpose of measuring electrical conductivity of the skin, an index called EDC (electrodermal conductance). It may be recalled that indicators of ANS function, such as EDC and a correlated measure of ANS variability called GSR (galvanic skin response), are associated with anxiety, tension, and fear, common components of POSR (*see* Tables 3.1, 3.2, and 3.3).

Biofeedback Techniques for POSR[5, 17, 42]

Biofeedback training is briefly defined as an IVP (number 5 in Table 8.2) as: "Focus is upon teaching persons to control largely involuntary components of POSR, heart rate or body temperature for example, by providing cues as to changes in that response." It is also indicated in Table 8.2 that the processes involved in biofeedback are learning and operant conditioning. Stated more definitively, biofeedback is a method based upon the fundamental principle of operant or Skinnerian conditioning, which maintains that most somatic and some autonomic responses followed closely by a correlated outcome cue may become learned responses capable of being sustained for some time. In a biofeedback procedure, involving learning to control such smooth muscle response as heart rate and blood pressure, for example, the exact nature of the subject's conditioning response is unknown. Some respondents describe their activity as a kind of psychoimagery, developing, for example, an image of a calm ocean, a brilliant sunset, or an auditory "image" of a Strauss waltz. Others describe the response as a "blotting out of all perceptions, a *tabula rasa*, a blank tablet." It is known that the simultaneous induction of a TRS as described in the discussion of the MPTRP above will effect a change in these conditioning responses in a biofeedback setting. The associated outcome cue or RF is usually a visual or auditory stimulus, an on/off colored light or buzzer, for instance. The time sequence for the introduction of the RF in modern-day biofeedback training is controlled by sensitive electronic circuitry designed to bring in the RF (the cue) *only* when the response meets the criterion programmed into the apparatus. For example, in treating tachycardia (fast pulse), a common aspect of POSR, a green light could be programmed to come on only when the pulse drops five or more bpm and a red light to come on when the rate increases five or more bpm. The same general sequence of events might be programmed to occur when treating hypertension, the criterion being a drop of ten or more mm Hg for the RF, a perceptible cue of any kind, to occur.

The literature pertaining to the success rates of biofeedback applied to cases of tachycardia, hypertension, tension headaches, and so on tends to support the general principle that most persons, some more effectively than others, can to some degree learn to control heart rate, blood pressure, skin temperature, and localized muscle tension, an example of the latter being the reduction in the jaw muscle tension, which causes the painful TMS (Temporomandibular Syndrome). However, as mentioned earlier, the exact nature of the processes by which these heretofore involuntary functions become voluntarily controlled through the learning processes involved in biofeedback remains unclear.

Although the response mechanisms are obscure, since 1962 the topic of biofeedback training to produce alpha brain waves has received a great deal of attention in the stress literature[60]. For example, it has been clearly demonstrated that most people, particularly musicians and other artists, can readily produce alpha rhythms by developing a relaxed, blank, inattentive, but awake state. The reinforcing cue most often used for this paradigm is a soft tone. As long as the tone sounds, alpha is sustained and, concomitantly, most subjects report a kind of calmness associated with a refreshed, comfortable frame of mind. These commonly reported subjective experiences occurring while alpha is being induced suggest the possibility that alpha wave generation may serve a function in POSR reduction and, by extension, in the enhancement of SCC.

Since a variety of electronically simple, inexpensive alpha generators have been on the market for some time, it comes as no surprise that a plethora of largely unsubstantiated claims pertaining to the beneficial effects of alpha induction have been publicized. For instance, it has been claimed that efficiency in learning new verbal material is increased while alpha is being elicited. It has been suggested that this improved learning rate may be the result in the reduction in general anxiety level during the alpha experience. Also, it has been reported that certain speech defects, such as stuttering, are alleviated or disappear altogether while alpha rhythms are sustained. Finally, some alpha enthusiasts have speculated that the pleasant "alpha high" may, in some cases, have the potential to substitute for the "high" induced by the ingestion of certain addictive drugs (stimulants and psychomimetic drugs, for example). Assuming that future research tends to verify these findings, it may be within the realm of possibility that alpha training may, to an extent, replace some of the psychotropic drugs presently being prescribed to control POSR[42].

Biofeedback involving changes in muscle potential as signalled by EMG tracings has been shown to be a useful IVP for some of the components of POSR, particularly for those symptoms resulting from long exposure to a high-SEP environment. For example, biofeedback techniques have been applied to the treatment of the often debilitating tension headaches, the etiology of which has been associated with chronic stress-inducing situations. One treatment program involves EMG tracings obtained from electrodes attached to the frontalis muscle of the forehead. In the training sessions, the subject is simply asked, "to remove as much of the tension from your forehead as you can . . . More! . . . More! . . . ." Similar to the schedule described above for the treatment of tachycardia, one common output cue sequence used in the treatment of tension headaches is to program the EMG synthesizer in such a way that a red light increases in brightness proportionate to the increase in the frequency and voltage of the EMG impulses, for example, gains in frequency from 20 to 100 cps and/or an increase in voltage in the range of 75 to 850 mv. As soon as the voltage drops below 375 mv, for example, and/or the frequency reaches a level below 20 cps, a green light replaces the red one. At this point, the subject is encouraged to "keep the green light on, do not let the red light come back on . . . make the green light brighter . . . brighter . . . brighter . . . ." The brighter the green light, the closer the electrical impulses from the muscle are approaching the 5 to 8 cps frequency range and/or the voltage is approaching the 300-mv level. After a relatively few training sessions, most headache sufferers are able, with minimal supervision, to carry out the biofeedback procedure each time the symptoms of tension headache become annoying, thus, in most cases, preventing the symptoms from becoming debilitating later on.

The literature reporting the results of the application of biofeedback for the treatment of tension headaches is generally favorable. Apparently, most patients can learn to reduce the muscular tension in the forehead to a level at or below the EMG criterion described above with a minimum of practice and in a matter of minutes. Most importantly, the majority of tension headache sufferers reports mitigation and sometimes complete remission of the most acute pain after three or four treatment sessions. Unfortunately, however, almost all of the patients report reoccurrence of acute episodes from time to time, indicating, of course, that biofeedback treatment functions as a control technique and not in any way as a cure[42].

Tables 3.2 and 3.3 and the correlated text in Chapter 3 describe the ANS component of POSR in some detail. As alluded to previously, one sensitive measure of the reactivity of the sympathetic branch of the ANS as it relates to anxiety and fear is the EDC, a measure of the electrical conductivity of the skin. A correlated measure is the GSR, an index of the variability of EDC. A person exposed to a high-SEP stressor (a sudden loud, unexpected noise, for example) would characteristically show an abrupt increase in EDC in the range of twenty-five to fifty micromhos conductance. As described in Chapter 3, this increase in EDC is correlated monotonically with sweat gland activity energized by the SNS. There are a number of reasonably efficient, inexpensive instruments that can be used to measure EDC, most effectively by means of electrodes placed in the palm of the hand. One example of this kind of equipment readily available to the layperson is a small gadget featuring a Wheatstone Bridge feedback loop that provides a fairly sensitive indication of changes in EDC. These changes are signaled by some output cue, usually an auditory tone of varying pitch. The lower the pitch of the output tone, the lower the EDC, indicative of a reduced tension or arousal level. Conversely, the higher the pitch of the tone, the greater the EDC and the correlated tension level. Accordingly, in order to reduce the subjective tension level, the person needs only to keep the tone at a very low pitch, lower . . . lower. . . . In fact, many of these gadgets are programmed for the tone to become inaudible when a maximum TRS is reached. In sum, this simple do-it-yourself biofeedback instrument provides a means by which anyone can reduce her/his tension and arousal level as needed to control the intensity of POSR.

Although the literature dealing with EDC and GSR as measures used in the lie detection procedure is quite copious, scientific studies of the efficacy of biofeedback involving control of EDC as a means of POSR reduction are sparse and out of date. However, the fact that the U.S. submarine service at one time issued "biofeedback cards" available on a voluntary basis for the submarine crewmembers suggests confidence that this technique may be helpful during long submerged missions. The wallet-size stress control card contains a small patch of hygroscopic (moisture-absorbing) substance, which, with thumb pressed firmly upon it for the count of ten, will change color from black (stressed) to red (tense) to green (normal) to blue (calm) (*see* reference 6). The color-change mechanism acts as an analogue of electrodermal sweating, and, in turn, of the activity of the SNS/anxiety-tension functional relationship. On the reverse side of the stress card are brief instructions prescribing relaxation techniques for reducing tension and other components of POSR.

9
Methodological Innovations for Stress Research

SCIENTIFIC METHOD AND POSR

One of the avant-garde of twentieth century American psychology, Dr. Walter Miles, once told the author that insofar as choice of subject matter is concerned, the scientific community reminded him of a termite-infested log. "How are scientists in their laboratories like termites?" I asked. "Termites (the scientists) vigorously attack the new wood in a log until a hole begins to appear (the growth of scientific knowledge). As the hole continues to expand, they begin to look for more new wood into which they start chewing again—the end result being several fairly intact logs dotted with holes of varying sizes and shapes, some overlapping and some clearly separated," was Dr. Miles' reply. As will be seen, this simile fits researchers in the area of stress very well.

What makes scientists periodically refocus their interests and research effort? An old time-worn story called the "drunkard's paradox" answers the question pointedly. This story goes: in the wee hours of the morning, a very inebriated drunk, on his hands and knees, crawling, falling, cursing, feeling with his hands in the grass surrounding a light post along a pathway in Central Park, was confronted by an Irish cop who asked, half jokingly, "Hey buddy, what are you doing crawling around this light post? Have you lost something?" Somewhat slurred, but trying desperately to demonstrate some degree of sobriety, the drunk, still in his crawling position, looking up at the cop, said, "Yeah! I lost my watch." "Where did you lose your watch?" the cop asked. "Over there in the bushes," was the quick reply. With a tone of disbelief, the cop asked, "Why the hell are you looking for it here under the light post if you lost it over there in the bushes?" "*This is where the light is*" was the drunk's unhesitating reply, as if to imply: Why do you ask?

So, throughout the history of science, researchers have characteristically been led in directions dictated by which "methodological lights" appear to be the brightest at the time. That is, they have tended to focus on those phenomena or subject matter areas that are most amenable for study by means of the methods or techniques that were available at that stage of history. Galileo studied the cosmos because the telescope was there. Similarly, Pasteur focused (no pun intended) on microorganisms as possible pathogens because Zacharias Janssen's sixteenth-century microscope was accessible. A more modern example of this trend in the history of science was the discovery by the nineteenth-century civil service worker and inventor Harry Hollerith of a system for representing alphanumeric data by punching holes in a card. This system, using Hollerith cards, became the forerunner for the "bit" or binary digit (a "0" or "1," a hole or no hole in the punched card), and ultimately became the basis for the present-day binary number system or code. In the past three decades, one needs no reminder of the phenomenal breakthroughs and spin-offs that have occurred in engineering, education, medicine, military technology (Desert Storm), and astronautics (*Apollo* and the moon) as the direct or indirect result of computer research and development based upon Hollerith's methodological insights.

Another lesson having to do with the major purpose of science may be inferred from the "drunkard's paradox" anecdote. That is, the purpose of science is *not* to use the light post as a disequilibrated, wobbly drunk might use it, for *support*, but rather to use the light on the post as it is meant to be used, for *illumination*, so that the surroundings can be seen more clearly—and, for science, the world around us can be better understood.

To elaborate on the last point, the goals of science are threefold: first, to contribute to a body of knowledge regarding the causes and consequences of events and phenomena around us; second, based upon the nature of the scientific method itself, to develop a frame of reference for understanding and predicting environmental occurrences, day-in-and-day-out, and, last, to develop the attitudes that many, if not most, of the severe problems related to human survival (wars, political unrest, and pestilence, for example) are caused by a variety of factors, most of which are identifiable by the scientific method.

There are, however, serious limitations resulting from the three philosophical assumptions underlying the scientific method itself: (1) *determinism*—if, by means of our ten sensory modalities we can ascertain that an event "Y" has occurred, it must be assumed that "Y" was caused by one or more equally observable variables, X_1, X_2; (2) *empiricism*—as implied in (1) above, the data of science is limited to observable, palpable information describable in terms of sensory input; and (3) *testability*—that is, the interrelationships between the independent variable(s) "X" and the dependent variable(s) "Y" as symbolized by the algebraic equation $Y = f(X)$ must be testable by the experimental methodology unique to science. The scientist does not study the phenomena of interest directly, but, instead, makes inferences about these phenomena from observable data. For example, temperature is *inferred* from the expansion or contraction of mercury in a tube, and the acid-base balance of a solution is likewise *inferred* from color changes in litmus paper. The observable data from which these inferences arise are called operational definitions of the phenomena in question. For instance, certain combinations of the variables in Table 3.3 become the operational definition of stress, or POSR. The validity and reliability of these operational definitions become still a fourth limitation of the scientific method. In sum, the scientific method symbolized by the equation above may be stated simply as the scientist's *modus operandi*: The scientist systematically manipulates the independent variable(s) and observes and measures the concomitant or consequent effects of this manipulation upon the dependent variable(s).

The purpose of this discussion of the general principles of the scientific method is to indicate the constraints upon the kinds of research possible in the area of stress. Now, with these constraints in mind, let us indicate the major directions research in this area might take. These directions or focal points can be epitomized in a three-word expression: what, how, and why? *What* variables, singly or in interactional relationships, are most and least highly correlated with stress reactivity, POSR? *How*, by what methods and techniques, can these variable interrelationships be most effectively analyzed and interpreted? *Why* do the multiplicity of variables, related in one way or another to POSR, interact as they do with numerous environmental stressors, frequently found in complex patterns? To summarize the three-word expression, is it possible to develop a theoretical model that provides a comprehensive frame of reference for interpreting the voluminous pool of data presently contained in the stress literature? Although perhaps arguable, the rationale for writing this book is that the ABC model of stress is at least a first start in fulfilling the requirements for a comprehensive frame of reference for interpreting stress data. At least "ABC" yields some insights into the "what" and "why" of the three-word summation. The "how" of that statement is the reason for this chapter. Furthermore, the first step in selecting the most appropriate methodology for research in any area is to ask the right research question(s) and in the right way. This matter is addressed next.

EVALUATION OF RESEARCH PROPOSALS ON STRESS

Most of the information on methodological issues in stress research found in this text is based upon findings emanating from the submarine literature dealing with various aspects of the topic of stress. One of the reasons for this emphasis on the submarine literature is that most of the R&D (research and development) proposals related to stress were screened by a specialized systematic evaluation procedure. The assumption was made that this thorough screening process applied to research proposals contributed significantly to the quality of the data originating from this source.

The R&D proposal evaluation form used in the past by some submarine researchers is presented in Appendix J. There are several unique features of this R&D proposal evaluation system used at one time by the Personnel Research Branch of the U.S. Naval Submarine Research Laboratory: first, ratings by qualified judges as to the degree to which the proposed research focuses on an isolatable hypothesis or research question associated with an applied problem critical for the success of submarine missions (criterion class I, Criticality and Focus; *see* Appendix J); second, criterion class II, Feasibility, requires the raters to indicate the likelihood that the appropriate laboratory equipment, the hardware and software for data analysis, and the opportunities to obtain representative subject samples from the population of concern are available; finally, criterion class III, Outcomes, requires probability estimates as to whether the results of the study will yield a definitive test of the research question(s) as posed, will have a significant applied value for the submarine service, and will make a substantive contribution to the fund of knowledge within the scientific community at large.

In practice, three or four experienced researcher-judges independently study each proposal after which she/he checks a point on each of the nine percentage scales to indicate the probability that each of the criterion subscales are in fact valid for the particular research proposal under consideration. Customarily, as indicated on the proposal evaluation form in Appendix J, an average probability value across the three criterion classes (nine criterion subscales in total) is calculated for each of the expert judges making the evaluations. Interrater agreement is usually examined for each of the nine criterion scales. In addition, weeks later, the same experts generally conduct a second evaluation of the proposal in order to ascertain further the reliability of their judgments.

FACTOR ANALYSIS AND STRESS RESEARCH

Leon Thurstone, one of the pioneers in the development of factor analytical methodology in the 1930's, described factor analysis as an extension of the correlational method aimed at the identification and interpretation of the major processes accounting for variable interaction. These processes or reference axes as Thurstone referred to them were symbolized by trigonometric vectors described in his book, *Vectors of the Mind*, as basic dimensions of personality[119]. In practice, these vectors or factors are generally rotated geometrically directly into clusters of variables plotted in a hypersphere (*see* Glossary) so as to simplify their interpretation. Thurstone called such a rotated solution "simple structure."

Other factor analysts simply describe factor analysis as a method for separating variables into those that are important (valid) and those that are unimportant (invalid) based upon their interrelationships, or, as a wheat farmer might describe the method, "it is one way of separating the wheat from the chaff"[41, 118].

At a more technical level, there are two broad objectives of factor analysis. One objective is to delineate and interpret the major dimensions or components underpinning a number of intercorrelated variables, which, since the advent of the computer era, may number as high as 200 or more. A second, less well-recognized objective of the factor analytical method, in particular as a methodological approach for stress research, is one of "hypothesis generation" and hypothesis testing[22, 130].

In reference to the what/how/why triad of foci in stress research discussed earlier, factor analysis addresses all of the three questions. That is, *what* variables are relevant, *how* can the variable interactions be most effectively delineated, and *why* do the particular processes underpinning the dimensions (factors) extracted by factor analysis of stress data interact in such a way as to determine the structure of the factor?

The seven types of factor analyses contained in Figure 9.1 serve both the function of dimension identification in some stress studies, and hypothesis generation and testing in others. Indeed, all of the seven types of factor analyses address in one way or another the three research questions epitomized in the what/how/why triad.

Before expanding on the unique characteristics of each of the seven types of factor analyses represented by the rectangular solid in Figure 9.1, certain aspects of the make-up of the figure itself should be addressed. Note, for example, that the combined term tests/measures, appearing as the horizontal dimension in the solid and also in the second column of the table, is shortened to "tests" elsewhere only to save space. Furthermore, it should be understood that tests/measures includes not only scores from paper and pencil tests but also may include scores from apparatus tests as well as indicators of psychophysiological processes. Finally, some of the column headings in the tabled section of the figure should be explained. Thus, the column headed "correlations between" refers to the three classes of variables (persons, tests/measures, and occasions) between which the correlation statistics are calculated. "Arrays over," the same expression as "distributions over," refers to the one of the three classes of variables making up the distributions of replicates between which the correlation coefficients are calculated. "Hold constant" pertains to the one plane of the three in the solid rectangle in Figure 9.1 that represents the one variable that is not involved in the statistical calculations carried out for the specific type of factor analysis being implemented. "Loadings on" refers to the one of the three classes of variables to which the factor loadings or weights are attached. Factor loadings indicate the degree to which each test or other measure, person, or occasion contributes to the structural definition of each factor or reference axis emerging from the analysis. Finally, "factor scores for" pertains to a score calculated for each replicate in the distributions of the one variable (person, test/measure, occasion) between which the correlations are obtained. Factor scores are calculated by means of a so-called "specification equation" that may be derived for each replicate in the distributions of correlated variables across all of the factors emerging from the analysis. For example, it is seen in Figure 9.1 that factor scores may be derived for persons in R-technique, for tests/measures in Q-technique, for occasions in P-technique, and so on. A brief discussion including examples of the application of each of the seven types of factor analysis presented in Figure 9.1 follows.

Figure 9.1
Seven Types of Factor Analyses Used in Stress Research

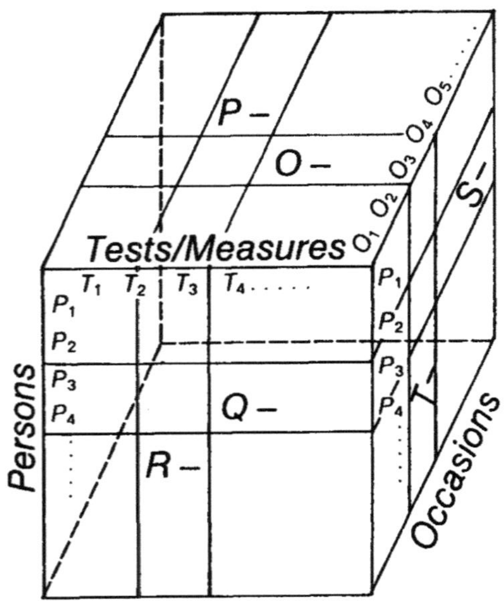

Technique	Correlations between	Arrays Over	Hold Constant	Loadings On	Factor Scores For
R-technique	tests/ measures	persons	occasions	tests	persons
Q-technique	persons	tests	occasions	persons	tests
P-technique	tests/ measures	occasions	one person	tests	occasions
O-technique	occasions	tests	one person	occasions	tests
T-technique	occasions	persons	tests	occasions	persons
S-technique	persons	occasions	tests	persons	occasions
Incremental R-technique	tests/ measures changes	persons	two occasions	test score changes	persons

R-Technique

R-technique is the most commonly used factor analytical strategy. As seen in Figure 9.1, scores from a number of tests or other measures are obtained from a sample of persons on one occasion or testing session. The structure of the factors is inferred from the content of the measures with high loadings on each factor. Also, the total test score variance (*see* Glossary) of each test/measure is accounted for by its loading pattern across all of the factors extracted in the analysis. Factors or dimensions defined by R-technique studies of stress-related topics generally represent underlying processes being measured by the matrix of tests/measures. R-factors, factors produced by R-technique studies in the stress area, identify the complex interactional dimensions of IED and AR resulting in POSR of varying degrees of intensity (*see* Equation 4.1).

One R-technique study involved the intercorrelations of fourteen measures of ANS responses resulting from a laboratory-induced, high-IED situation, three psychometric test scores (aptitude, anxiety, and motivation), and two performance criterion dimensions based upon supervisor ratings obtained during a forty day submerged mission. The data for the resulting 19 × 19 correlation matrix were obtained from 140 nuclear submariners. Emerging from the factor analysis of this matrix were five R-factors, tentatively labeled: F_1 (Factor 1), Limited Adjustment Potential; F_2, Optimal Adjustment Potential; F_3, Autonomic Recoverability; F_4, Autonomic Feedback; and F_5, Stress Reactivity[144].

How may the findings of this R-technique study be interpreted? F_1, Limited Adjustment Potential, was defined, that is, had high factor loadings, by two ANS indicators, namely, large skin resistance changes to two laboratory-contrived conflict situations. In contrast, F_2, Optimal Adjustment Potential, was defined by small skin resistance changes and by large increases in measures of autonomic recoverability following induced POSR. Taken together, the structures of F_1 and F_2 suggested the hypothesis that the quality of submariner adjustment is related to minimal change and high recoverability of the ANS of submariner candidates exposed to certain contrived high-IED conditions.

In sum, this R-technique factor analytical study of the stress reactivity of nuclear submariners yielded five dimensions or factors that may be interpreted as components of POSR. At the same time, several hypotheses pertaining to the relationship between ANS resiliency and the SCC of nuclear submariners were also generated.

Q-Technique

As indicated in Figure 9.1, Q-technique, sometimes called inverse or obverse factor analysis, involves the inverse of the R-technique correlation matrix[114, 129]. An inverse matrix in this case means that the rows (persons) in the R-technique matrix become the columns of the Q-technique correlation matrix. Thus, the correlational statistics are calculated between persons over arrays of traits, tests, or other measures obtained on one occasion. In Q-technique, factor loadings are derived for persons, and these patterns of loadings define the structure of the Q-factors.

Q-technique is frequently described as an empirical method for "typing" people. In Q-technique studies involving Q-sorts (*see* Glossary), the correlation matrix is derived from the intercorrelation of the arrays of traits, each listed on a Q-card and rank ordered by experts whose task is to describe the personalities of members of a specified population. The rank order continuum usually extends from "most" to "least" descriptive of the population of concern.

A unique example of the typing application of Q-technique is to be found in a study of the nine Supreme Court judges during the 1943–44 sessions[121]. The voting records of the nine justices considering each court case reaching the court during these sessions were ranked by legal scholars on the bipolar scale "tending toward conservatism or toward liberalism." The 9 × 9 correlation matrix was derived from between-judge phi coefficients (*see* Glossary) calculated between the arrays of voting records for each judge on the 115 cases considered during that time span. Three factors emerged, the major factor being identified by Justice Black and Justice Douglas, whose voting patterns suggested a strong liberal component within the Court at that time. Thus, Q-methodology was instrumental in identifying trait dimensions of persons within a judicial body whose decisions affect almost everyone of the U.S. populace in one way or another.

Just prior to the launching of the *Nautilus*, the first atomic submarine, in 1954, a Q-technique study was carried out to identify the predominant pattern or patterns of personality traits associated with individual differences in the SCC of nuclear submariners[129]. The Q-sorters consisted of seven submarine medical officers, six submarine line officers, and one civilian psychologist (the author). The trait battery, placed on Q-cards, consisted of seventy-eight descriptors obtained from a series of studies using the Critical Incident Technique (*see* Glossary), and was conducted with both officer and enlisted submarine personnel with many years of experience in the submarine service. Examples of these trait-descriptors placed on Q-cards are: cooperative, optimistic, realistic, enthusiastic, alert, and so on.

Three orthogonal (axes at 90°) factors emerged from the factor analysis of this 14 × 14 matrix of Q-sorts. However, only the first two factors, F_1 and F_2, significantly "loaded" by six and five officer-Q-sorters, respectively, were interpretable. Based upon the nature of the descriptors ranked highest and lowest as descriptive of an effective nuclear submariner, the F_1 "Q-type" of submariner had a high SCC by virtue of his having dominant traits related to emotional control. On the other hand, the SCC exemplified by the F_2 "Q-type" resulted from the presence of traits related to effective social skills.

Thus, these studies suggest that Q-methodology is useful in stress research when the central question is, "What pattern of traits is associated with individual differences in SCC?" With this information in hand, it is possible to identify persons with maximum AR for adjusting optimally to an environment with high IED.

P-Technique

Looking again at the rectangular solid in Figure 9.1, the uniqueness of P-technique (P for personal) and its inverse O-technique is that only *one* person is involved in the analysis[23]. Like R-technique, the correlation matrix for P-technique results from intercorrelating between a number of traits, test scores, or other measures obtained from one person repeatedly over an array of occasions. P-technique, therefore, yields P-factors defined by factor loadings on tests/measures as in R-technique. Further, factor scores may be calculated for each measurement session or occasion, the number of occasions being at least ten, but possibly as high as fifty or hundreds, or, with the modern computer technology available, in the thousands.

One P-technique study focused on individual differences in the SCC of three certified U.S. Navy divers [141]. A sustained high-IED environment resulted from the incarceration of the divers in a pressure chamber with an oxygen/nitrogen mixed gas atmosphere maintained at seven atmospheres absolute pressure, or about 103 PSI (pounds per square inch), for a duration of sixteen days. Five measures of the divers' adaptive state were obtained twice daily during the confinement period. The measures were: SRT (sequential reaction time), SRT-errors (or reactive response accuracy), and adjective checklist scores on anxiety, hostility, and depression. A 5 × 5 P-technique correlation matrix was derived for each diver, each diver's ten correlation coefficients having been calculated between tests over arrays of thirty-two occasions (sixteen days).

The P-technique correlation matrices for each diver together with the rotated factor matrices adjacent are presented in Table 9.1.

At the outset, attention should be called to "h^2" in the righthand column in Table 9.1. It refers to the communality of each of the five measures. The communality of a given measure differs from the reliability of that measure only by the amount of specific factor variance, a measure of the score variation due to the unique characteristics of the measure itself[41]. Therefore, the h^2 statistics in Table 9.1 provide an approximate estimate of the reliability of each measure involved in the factor analysis.

The data in Table 9.1 demonstrate the most important methodological use of P-technique in stress research, namely, to identify trend of fluctuation factors with respect to which a given individual's SCC may be assessed. In the study under discussion, for example, the CAP ("Characteristic Adaptive Pattern") of each of the three divers was deduced from his factor loading pattern presented in Table 9.1. A quote from the paper concerning Diver B's CAP demonstrates the methodological point to be made:

Table 9.1
Correlation Matrices and Rotated Factor Loadings for Three Diver-Subjects

Subject	Correlation Matrices					Rotated Factor Matrices		
A Measures	I	II	III	IV	V	F_1	F_2	h^2
I SRT						00	80	64
II SRT-errors	-28					-08	37	14
III Anxiety	36	-16				56	48	54
IV Hostility	-58	21	34			42	82	85
V Depression	15	-12	31	50		68	18	49
B Measures	I	II	III	IV	V	F_1	F_2	h^2
I SRT						70	16	52
II SRT-errors	-27					68	68	92
III Anxiety	41	25				63	-42	57
IV Hostility	-31	21	27			58	00	34
V Depression	56	-87	42	42		99	01	98
C Measures	I	II	III	IV	V	F_1	F_2	h^2
I SRT						-12	64	42
II SRT-errors	30					-12	60	37
III Anxiety	-17	-19				-14	88	79
IV Hostility	38	34	19			14	68	48
V Depression	14	16	82	31		18	98	99

Decimals are omitted. With N = 27–32 measurement sessions, a product-moment correlation coefficient of 0.36 is significant at the 5 percent level.

Source: Reference 141, p. 268. Copyright © 1978 by Undersea and Hyperbaric Medical Society, Inc. Reprinted by permission of Undersea and Hyperbaric Medical Society, Inc.

Subject B's characteristic adaptive pattern (CAP) stands out from those of the other divers largely by the high correlation of his depression score with the two performance measures and with the other two measures of affectivity. While this finding may be only coincidental, it is at least interesting and possibly heuristic that Subject B reported the most acute and prolonged symptoms of nausea the first 41 hours of the saturation phase of the experiment[141, p. 268].

There are several other methodological possibilities of P-technique in stress research, for example, for the treatment of stress disorders. In one study, P-technique was applied to a correlation matrix obtained from the covariance patterns of measures of general psychiatric status, such as endocrinological and psychophysiological indexes and measures of mood and emotional reactivity (POSR) repeatedly measured in one patient over a sequence of twenty therapy sessions[23]. The factors derived from this P-technique analysis provided insights into which processes (muscular tension for example) were and were not being affected by the therapeutic strategies being used. Also, one submarine study combined P-technique and Q-technique by first identifying personality types of submariners by Q-technique, and then investigating individual differences in the

SCC of each "Q-type" when exposed to the high-SEP stressors associated with sixty-days' confinement within a submarine[130]. The differences between the "Q-types" in terms of the structure of their P-technique trend or fluctuation factors obtained during the sixty-day incarceration were clearly delineated and readily interpretable as indexes of SCC.

Finally, there are several studies using a slight modification of the standard P-technique research design[151]. One such study in the literature of submarine stress was conducted during the 80-day submerged circumnavigation of the world by the submarine *Triton* in 1960[136]. This study involved the collection of self-ratings on fifty rating scales applied to fifty submariners. The scales were designed to measure mood, interpersonal attitudes, fatigue, and the like each day of the eighty-day mission. The correlation coefficients were calculated between the daily *average* scores for the fifty men on each of the fifty scales rather than between each *individual's* scores on each scale over arrays of eighty days (occasions), as is customarily done in P-technique. This modified P-technique study yielded two major factors. The factor loadings for the most important single factor are contained in Table 9.2.

Judging from the meanings of the descriptors with high factor loadings, this factor appears to be indicative of agitated depression, sadness, and frustration, all components of POSR[138]. If an average factor score for the fifty submariners is calculated for each day of the eighty-day mission, it is possible to identify the points in time during the submerged voyage that depressive trends and other POSR began to appear. The plot of these average factor scores is contained in Figure 9.2.

With the average factor scores correlated positively with the intensity of POSR, the peaks (greater intensity of POSR) and troughs (lesser intensity of POSR) in Figure 9.2 may be inspected for covariance with the occurrence of selected daily events. Although correlation does not necessarily mean causation, nonetheless the possibility exists that some of these mood and motivational fluctuations in the polygon in Figure 9.2 may have been, in part, caused by certain daily events.

One example of this causal relationship in Figure 9.2 is the continuous drop in the factor score curve, suggesting a similar drop in POSR from day sixty to the end of the trip, is immediately apparent. On the sixtieth day, while the *Triton* was in the Atlantic Ocean off Spain, information was inadvertently leaked that the submarine would surface off the Delaware Straits approximately two weeks hence. Psychologists call the apparent increase in overall morale indicated in the graph the "end effect" or "end spurt." British sailors noted the same phenomenon upon entering the English Channel when returning from a mission during World War II. They, quite appropriately, labeled this sequence of events "channel fever." The point is that subjective and other data plotted in factor score form over time provide useful insights into subtle changes in the intensity level of POSR.

Overall, P-technique, including the slight design variation seen in Figure 9.2, is effective in stress research as a methodological strategy for delineating some

Table 9.2
Factor Loadings for the Adjectives and Behavioral Statements Rated Daily during the World Circumnavigation of the Submarine *Triton*

Variable number	Loading[a]	Content[b]
7	.88	Morale low
22	.76	Fed up
10	.70	Irritable
37	.68	Homesick
15	.65	Don't feel like talking
13	.64	Annoyed
24	.64	Disinterested
41	.64	Feel like giving up
11	.63	Mouth dry
4	.59	Bored stiff
5	.58	Don't feel like doing anything
19	.58	Daydream a lot
40	.58	Headachy
43	.58	Uncomfortable
50	.56	Frustrated

[a]Factor has been reflected.

[b]Takes into account the sign of the loading.

Source: Reference 136, p. 106. Copyright © 1963 by The Free Press, a Division of Macmillan, Inc. Reprinted by permission of Macmillan Publishing Company.

of the major mechanisms associated with adapting to high-SEP stressors imposed over long periods of time.

O-Technique

From an examination of Figure 9.1, it is seen that O-technique is the inverse of P-technique. Although again only one person is involved, in O-technique the correlations are obtained between occasions over arrays of tests/measures rather than between tests/measures over arrays of occasions, as in "P." Insofar as the usefulness of O-technique as compared to P-technique in stress research is concerned, "P," a *personal* design strategy, yields an assessment of one person's SCC in terms of changes in adaptive processes over a series of changes in IED referred to as "occasions." P-factors describe a person's AR to sequentially introduced stressors. On the other hand, O-technique, a *psychoecological* design strategy, delineates dimensions derived from the patterns of factor loading of changes in the IED associated with different environmental conditions called occasions. Stated differently, O-factors serve to identify communalities of environmental dimensions across varying IED's. In short, P-technique focuses on

Figure 9.2
Plot of the Factor Scores for the Eighty-Day Global Circumnavigation of the *Triton*

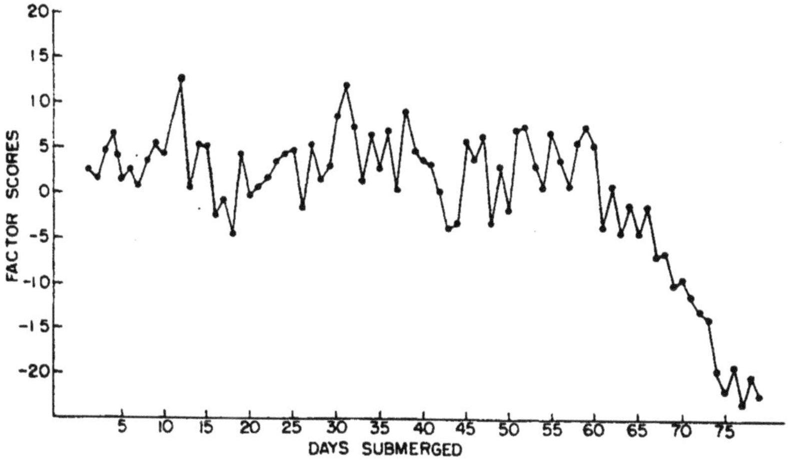

Source: Reference 136, p. 107. Copyright © 1963 by The Free Press, a Division of Macmillan, Inc. Reprinted by permission of Macmillan Publishing Company.

the one person, whereas O-technique focuses on the environment of that one person.

Insofar as is known, there are no published studies demonstrating the use of O-technique in stress research. However, dating back to the 1940's, there were a number of psychoecological studies in which several environmental dimensions were intercorrelated, the purpose being to identify communalities in the environment accounting for selected behaviors. O-technique, consisting of factor analyzing these correlation matrices separately for individuals (those presenting different POSR for example), could have conceivably produced important, heretofore unknown, environmental dimensions (O-factors) associated with individual differences in the SCC to these kinds of stressors[22].

At present, the methodological possibilities of O-technique for research in the stress area are considerable. As this section of the book is being written, Operation Desert Shield is at a crisis point. Without question, the IED on a day-to-day basis is very high for the majority of the men and women of the military forces deployed in that region of the Middle East. O-technique could be effectively applied to several research questions related to stress reactivity (POSR) that have already been raised during this campaign. For example, one frequently posed question has to do with possible differences in the SCC of men and women in this high-IED desert environment. An O-technique study to shed some light on this question might start with drawing random samples of six or more military personnel of each sex from the population at risk, being careful to equate the individuals in the samples for branch of service, rank/rate, age, time in service, and all other pertinent variables that can be held constant. Scores on thirty or so psychophysiological and personality measures as well as three or four adjustment criterion scores could be collected from each person in both samples during two time intervals: every three weeks during the four months' basic training prior to deployment and the same measures every three weeks during the first four months' deployment in the desert. With each of the thirty scores for each of the twelve persons in standard score form, a 10 × 10 correlation matrix could then be developed *for each person* with five predeployment measurement sessions (occasions) and five postdeployment sessions making up the columns, and the thirty personality and other scores making up the rows of the correlation matrices.

A comparison of the structure of the factors extracted by "O" factor analysis of each of the twelve matrices, one for each military person, will delineate the major processes associated with the similarity and differences in SCC within and between sexes at two levels of IED, namely, predeployment training and postdeployment field training, in preparation for war.

However, the comparisons of the SCC of men and women in this hypothetical study will of course be limited by the nature of the thirty test/measurement and criterion scores selected for the study. As in P-technique, yet another rather obvious limitation of any O-technique study is the restriction of subject sampling to only *one* person. In spite of these limitations, "O" will yield factor scores that identify the measure or measures that interact most and least with each IED condition (pre- versus postdeployment in the above example) for each person of both sexes in the subject samples. The between-person variation in the one or more tests or other measures identified by O-technique can then be examined by an analogue of "O," T-technique, to be discussed below.

T-Technique

T-technique consists of factor analyzing a group of test-retest reliability coefficients (r_{tt}) for *one* test or other measure over arrays of the same persons on two or more occasions[22]. Since the factors extracted by T-technique will be "loaded" (have factor loadings) on occasions, the factor structure will be characterized by clusters of occasions that, in stress research, will describe differences and similarities in stressor patterns across a number of occasions (*see* Figure 9.1). Stated differently, the T-factor structure will indicate the degree to which different IED's affect the performance on the one measure being considered. Since factor loading patterns are by occasions, T-technique is similar to O-technique, except that in "O" the concern is for *one* person, whereas in "T" a *distribution* of persons is involved.

As before, there are no known published studies using the T-technique design in the literature of stress at this time. Yet, again, there are several methodological possibilities for the use of "T" to investigate various aspects of stress. For example, the indirect measurement of arterial blood pressure by the familiar auscultatory method is often used in studies of POSR in spite of the well-known fact that this technique lacks acceptable reliability, or, as the statistician would say, blood pressure measurements obtained by this method have very large error variance. Some of the major sources of error are: positioning of the pressure cuff on the arm, left or right arm, the type of auditory sensor diaphragm, the training level of the technician and his/her auditory acuity, physical and emotional condition of the patient and technician, postprandial time of the patient, and so on.

The application of the T-technique design to the problem of identifying and weighing the main error dimensions in the distributions of a sample of blood pressure readings obtained by this method is straightforward. First, consider the hypothetical sources of error to be the "occasions" in T-technique. For example, O_1 (occasion 1) might be cuff placed high on the upper left arm; O_2, cuff placed *low* on the same arm; O_3, experienced technician; O_4, inexperienced; O_5, no meal; O_6, meal before measurement; and so on. Since the computer hardware and software necessary to conduct factor analyses of huge correlation matrices in nanoseconds are readily available, the number of occasions (i.e., experimental conditions) can be very large indeed. Recall, however, if "n" equals the number of occasions, then the number of different *pairs* of occasions to be correlated is given by the simple formula $(n-1)\ n/2$—for instance, a 4×4 matrix would require the calculation of 6 coefficients, whereas a 16×16 matrix would require 120 calculations, and so on. For the proposed experiment ($n=6$), the fifteen correlations between distributions of blood pressure readings obtained for each occasion from samples of thirty, fifty, or more persons could then be developed into a 6×6 correlation matrix for T-technique factorization. The structure of the T-factors defined by patterns of factor loadings on occasions (hypothetical sources of measurement error in this study) should delineate and weigh the major error dimensions affecting the accuracy of blood pressure data obtained by the auscultatory method.

Finally, there is one additional methodological use of T-technique in many scientific studies, those dealing with stress included. This use of "T," purely a statistical use, would be to obtain an accurate estimate of the reliability of one person's score on a specific test or other measure in a number of IED situations of varying intensities. For example, let us consider the calculation of a correlation matrix required for the implementation of T-technique with the D-scale (Depression Scale) of the MMPI (Minnesota Multiphasic Personality Inventory). The MMPI would be administered to the same population sample (N = 1,000 or more) on ten successive occasions separated by equal time intervals and with each occasion representing different IED levels. Upon calculation of the reliability coefficients between all pairs of "occasions," forty-five in all, a 10×10

matrix would result, and a T-technique factor analysis could then be conducted. The T-factor structure would indicate in which of the ten occasions (IED levels) the D-scale is most and least reliable.

At this point, it may be well to indicate an important statistical spin-off resulting from the development of the "T" correlation matrix itself[47]. A very important statistic, the SEM (standard error of measurement), can be calculated for each of the forty-five test-retest coefficients (r_{tt}) in the example cited above by the formula: $SEM = SD_D (1 - r_{tt})^{1/2}$ where, SD_D is the standard deviation of the D-scale distribution used in the example, and r_{tt} equals the test/retest reliability between any pair of the forty-five coefficients. To demonstrate the use of the SEM statistic, let us assume that a male adult earned a raw score of seventeen on the D-scale, which, in this hypothetical sample, had an SD of five raw score units, and one of the reliability coefficients (r_{tt}'s) (e.g. between O_1 and O_6) was 0.64. Substituting these data in the formula for SEM, $SEM = 5 (1 - 0.64)^{1/2}$, we find SEM = 3 raw score units. The interpretation of this finding is important and, indeed, quite simple. With SEM = 3, the so-called 99 percent confidence interval or confidence span for this one man's D-score of seventeen would be $17 \pm 2.58(3)$ or about 9.3 to 24.7. Translated, the odds are 99 percent that, upon retesting with the D-scale of the MMPI, this man's true score will lie between 9.3 and 24.7 units on the D-scale. The same calculation can of course be carried out for the remaining forty-four r_{tt}'s, thus providing important information pertaining to fluctuations in the reliability of a given test or other measure as environmental conditions (occasions in the "T" analysis) vary. Obviously, test construction experts generally strive to maximize the r_{tt} of their tests, since it is noted in the formula for SEM that, as r_{tt} approaches unity, the magnitude of the SEM approaches zero, indicating errorless measurement.

In sum, in addition to delineating the major dimensions of error (i.e., the T-factors) for a given test or other measure, the correlation matrix required for a T-technique factor analysis also yields a very useful measure of the accuracy of a given person's raw score on that same test or measure. Finally, since the columns of the correlation matrix basic to "T" are occasions, the possibilities for systematically varying these experimental conditions or occasions (IED levels, for example) in order to determine the resulting changes in the T-factor structure are enormous and indeed challenging.

S-Technique

S-technique, requiring the calculation of the inverse correlation matrix used in T-technique, is similarly concerned with scores on only *one* test or other measure[22]. The measurement scores are obtained from two to twenty or more persons on a sizable number of occasions. Like Q-technique, the correlational statistics are calculated in S-technique between persons, but the arrays of replicates consist of occasions rather than test/measures. Q- and S-techniques are also similar in that factor loadings are derived for persons (*see* Figure 9.1).

Again, insofar as is known, there are no published studies using the S-technique design in the literature of stress emanating either from the submarine service or elsewhere. As before, however, there are a number of research possibilities. Since only one kind of measurement datum, is required, the S-technique strategy makes possible the manipulation of environmental stressors in such a manner that the occasions, say twenty or more, are at different IED levels, either localized in the field or contrived in the laboratory. Thus, factor scores may be derived for each occasion or IED level, and, since the structure of the S-factors is a function of the "loading" patterns of persons, it is possible to ascertain which person is most and least likely to have adequate SCC to adapt optimally to each IED level.

A hypothetical example of the application of S-technique to a stress situation could come from one aspect of the submariner screening program. Until recently, all submariner candidates were required to pass the CCT (compression chamber test)[141]. The CCT consisted of locking the submariner candidates in groups of twelve to fifteen in a compression chamber. One purpose of the CCT was to screen for claustrophobic tendencies. The CCT procedure consisted of gradually increasing the air pressure to about three atmospheres relative pressure, or about forty-five PSI. As the pressure increased from standard pressure (fifteen PSI) to forty-five PSI, the heat, the high-frequency noise of the air entering the chamber, and, in some cases, the pain of a ruptured eardrum caused about 10 to 15 percent of the candidates to say "uncle" and ask to be removed from the chamber before maximum pressure was reached. Voluntary removal from the chamber before reaching forty-five PSI pressure disqualified the candidate for submarine duty.

To apply the S-technique to the CCT situation, one could test the hypothesis that the capacity to tolerate high air pressure is a function of the amount of experience submariner candidates have had in pressurized air. Stepwise, such an experiment could be implemented as follows: First, randomly assign four groups of submariner candidates, three men in each group, to four levels of training in pressurized air. Group A (G-A) would receive *no* training, G-B would do *three* "dives" (simulated dives in a pressure chamber) to two atmospheres pressure (thirty PSI), G-C would do *six* dives to the same maximum pressure, and G-D would do *nine* dives to that pressure. Second, following this training phase, heart rate data would be obtained from each of the twelve subjects while at standard pressure. Third, the experimental phase of the study would begin by subjecting all twelve subjects to thirty-one consecutive "dives." Carrying out two "dives" daily, A.M. and P.M., the chamber air pressure would start at standard pressure for the first "dive," increasing 0.1 atmospheres (1.5 PSI) for the next thirty exposures until three atmospheres pressure is reached during the thirty-first "dive," or, stated in the language of S-technique, the sequence could be described as a series of thirty-one successive "occasions," each occasion representing graduated increases in IED caused by increasing pressure. Obviously, precise measures of the dependent variable, in this experiment, heart rate, would be obtained from each of the twelve subjects during each of the thirty-one "dives." Fourth and finally, calculate the 12 × 12 between-person, over-thirty-one-occasions correlation matrix of heart rate data, and conduct an S-technique factor analysis.

Assuming that differences in heart rate data are valid measures of individual differences in the intensity of POSR in submariner candidates, the structure of the S-factors defined by the loading patterns of the nontrained as compared with those subjects with different amounts of training in pressurized air should clearly indicate the effectiveness of this kind of training upon the SCC of submariner candidates.

Extrapolations from this hypothetical example of the application of S-technique suggest other challenging research possibilities in such critical social areas as drug abuse and AIDS prevention, to name two such areas. For instance, in the pressurization experiment presented above, suppose that six to eight randomized, small groups of preadolescents, ages from 9 to 13 of both sexes, were substituted for the submariner training groups, and these young persons were given different amounts of drug education. One group, acting as a control, would of course receive no drug education. Instead of heart rate as the dependent variable, the experimental variable might be the frequency of drug-related violations during a specified time frame. The "occasions" could be four-month intervals during which infractions would be recorded for each subject instead of the heart rate data collected for each subject during each of the thirty-one "dives" in the earlier experiment. The data collection for the drug experiment might continue for six years, thus yielding a total of eighteen occasions.

Upon S-technique factorization of the correlation matrix obtained from correlating between-persons over arrays of occasions (four-month intervals), some insights into several pertinent questions are possible: at what age is drug education most effective; is there a sex difference in the effectiveness of drug education, and at what age does this difference become most apparent; and, are there recidivistic trends in the data over time, and, if so, at what age does this recidivism appear?

The reader is encouraged to extrapolate the S-technique strategies described in the two experiments outlined above to a number of situations and conditions related to stress reactivity. Having done this, the scientific power of the S-technique design will most likely be more fully appreciated.

Incremental R-Technique

IRT (Incremental R-technique) is considered by some stress researchers to be the most powerful multivariate research design for the identification of the trend and fluctuation dimensions of POSR. Moreover, the assumptions underpinning IRT are consistent with those assumptions basic to the ABC model of stress (*see* Figure 3.1). To reiterate, these assumptions are (1) stress, that is POSR (patterns of stress reactivity) refers to dynamic (vice static) multivariate reactions to immediately perceived or anticipated blockage of goal-directed behavioral contingencies, and (2) to be meaningful, studies of the nature of the components of POSR (Table 3.3) must focus less upon baseline or prestress data and more upon the patterns of measures of *changes* in reactivity resulting from the intrusion of environmental blockages called stressors.

Accordingly, IRT focuses upon *patterns of change-processes* occurring before and after exposure to one or more high-SEP stressors. Similar to the static R-technique design discussed earlier, in IRT, the dynamic R-technique, the correlation coefficients are calculated between 20 to 200 or more tests/measures over arrays of persons. In regular "R," however, the measures are obtained under static baseline or prestress conditions, whereas in IRT, the focus is upon the measurement of change-scores consisting of *differences* between pre- and poststress scores on all variables included in the study. As seen in Figure 9.1, the factor structure in IRT is defined by loading patterns of *changes* (poststress to prestress) in the tests or other measures making up the study. Since, in IRT, factor scores may be calculated for persons, it is possible to derive predictive equations between a person's SCC defined by patterns of *change-scores* and selected adaptive criteria associated with different IED levels.

There are only two known publications in which the IRT design was used primarily to extract the change or fluctuation dimensions (factors) describing individual differences in SCC to elevated IED situations[132, 148]. The first study involved obtaining eighteen autonomic and behavioral measures before and after a contrived high-IED scenario was introduced. The subjects were eighty-one candidates being screened for guard positions in a state prison. The stress induction procedure consisted of abruptly blocking the candidates' attempts to erect a tent on the prison grounds while being observed by several trained psychologists, dressed as prison guards. The IRT was applied to the 18 × 18 correlation matrix constructed by correlating between the eighteen change-scores (poststress minus prestress), which had been transformed to standard (Z-score) units (*see* Glossary). The rotated factor solution yielded two well-defined ANS change factors, one a sympathetic nervous system dimension and the other a parasympathetic nervous system dimension. Factor scores calculated for the eighty-one subjects correlated significantly with the Army General Classification Test and with scores on the Cornell Selectee Index, measures of verbal aptitude and neurotic symptoms, respectively.

The statement in the above paragraph that the change-scores were transformed to Z-score units raises a methodological problem unique to any stress research involving analysis of change-score data. The problem, called the LIV (Law of Initial Value), refers to a common characteristic of change-score distributions[158]. Briefly, the LIV states, "there is a significant correlation (usually negative) between baseline or prestress measures of dependent variables and the change-scores (post-stress minus prestress) for the same variable." For example, person A with a prestress resting systolic blood pressure of 110 as compared to person B in the same subject sample with a pressure of 190 will likely show a greater poststress increase in systolic pressure than will person B because of the wide differences in their baseline levels. To reiterate, baseline or prestress scores tend to be negatively correlated with poststress change-scores. In the above example of the two persons with widely different baseline blood pressures, let us suppose that they both obtained the same change-scores (e.g., thirty mm Hg increase) following the high-IED exposure. The meaning of these two identical change-scores would quite likely be very different in terms of the cardiovascular dynamics underlying these changes. As a result, to be meaningful, a score transformation of some kind is needed to avoid the confounding of change-scores with their baseline or prestress levels.

Since this chapter focuses on methodology appropriate for research in the area of stress, this would seem to be the place to suggest approaches for correcting for the confounding effects of the LIV. The most simple and perhaps the most frequently used technique for reducing the LIV effect is to change the poststress scores to percentage gain or loss of the baseline or prestress levels[66]. However, a more elegant and statistically reliable technique for eliminating the LIV effect is called the "partitioning method," which, incidentally, was used in the IRT study presented above[132]. This method consists of four steps: (1) the baseline or prestress distributions for each dependent variable are dichotomized at the median resulting in an "upper" and a "lower" baseline group for each variable; (2) then, the means and SD's for the distributions of change-scores (poststress—baseline) for each variable is calculated separately for the "upper" and "lower" groups in the baseline distributions; (3) next, for each of the dependent variables, and still separately within the "upper" and "lower" groups, each person's change-score is transformed to a z-score (*see* Glossary); and finally, (4) in order to remove the negative z-scores, each change-score in z-score units is further changed to Z-scores by the simple equation, Z-score = 10z + 50. The resulting Z-score distribution of change-scores will then have a mean of fifty and a SD of ten. This series of score transformations allows for the calculation of the correlation matrix of change-scores irrespective of their baseline or prestress levels. In other words, the partitioning technique partials out the effect of the LIV.

A more recent example of a factor analytical study using the IRT design including the partitioning technique for controlling for LIV involved sixteen graduate student registrants in a university seminar devoted exclusively to the topic of stress[148]. The objectives of the study were to delineate the major affective components of POSR resulting from the exposure of graduate students to a high-IED situation. The dependent variables consisted of the thirty items of the ARI (Affective Response Inventory), a bipolar self-rating inventory designed to measure such aspects of POSR as afraid/unafraid, palms sweaty/palms dry, upset/calm, and so on. Although the ARI used in this experiment contained the same thirty bipolar items as the ARI in Appendix B, it did not include the timeline rating scale, an important aspect of the form in Appendix B. The instructions to the participants in this study were simply, "check the point on each of the thirty scales that describes yourself *now*, at the *present* time." The

ARI was administered before and after the introduction of a contrived high-IED situation. The stress induction procedure consisted of asking the students to first complete the ARI form in a calm, relaxed atmosphere. Then, after collecting the prestress ARI data, suddenly, and without warning an unannounced midterm test covering some of the most complex aspects of the stress literature was introduced. Examples of these threatening test items are: clearly differentiate between the peripheral indicators of PNS and SNS reactivity included in the concept of POSR, and compare and contrast the terms "psychosomatic" and "somatopsychic" in the context of POSR. After allowing ample time to deliberate over the difficult test and, at the same time, making sure that the students realized that their performance on the test was crucial for their final grade in the seminar, the subjects were again asked to complete another ARI form. After collecting the second ARI data, it was summarily announced that because of time constraints, it was decided to postpone the midterm examination for two weeks.

Following the application of the partitioning technique to the change-scores on each of the thirty items of the ARI, the 30 × 30 correlation matrix was developed and factor analyzed. Ten bipolar dimensions (factors) were extracted, the first three of which clearly identified the major affective dimensions describing the POSR of graduate students exposed to this particular high-IED situation. These three bipolar factors were tentatively labeled: reactive anxiety/unpleasant affect, tense anger/focused hostility, and depressed mood/anergia.

In sum, these two studies demonstrate the efficacy of the IRT of factor analysis to produce dimensions defining stress-induced patterns of changes in the processes making up the total POSR to particular stress situations. Further, it was demonstrated clearly that the change-score distributions, part-and-parcel of IRT, must be corrected for the so-called LIV effect. The "partitioning technique," described in detail in this section, is recommended for that purpose.

THE STAIR-STEPPING HYPOTHESIS

A monumental study of the U.S. Air Force pilots during World War II was conducted to assess the predictive validity of peripheral indexes of ANS function (Table 3.1) in relation to the quality of performance during training flights[128]. The data from this R-technique factor analytic study produced a dynamic concept labeled "Autonomic Balance," reflecting the homeostatic relationship between the parasympathetic and sympathetic branches of the ANS. Peripheral indexes of ANS balance turned out to be the most valid predictor of individual differences in pilot performance.

Extending these findings from the air force, coupled with related data bearing on the relationship of ANS resiliency and SCC from the submarine service, we developed and partially tested a related model that came to be called the "Stair-stepping Hypotheses"[137, 146]. A schematic representing this model is presented in Figure 9.3.

Figure 9.3
Schematic Representation of the Stair-Stepping Hypothesis

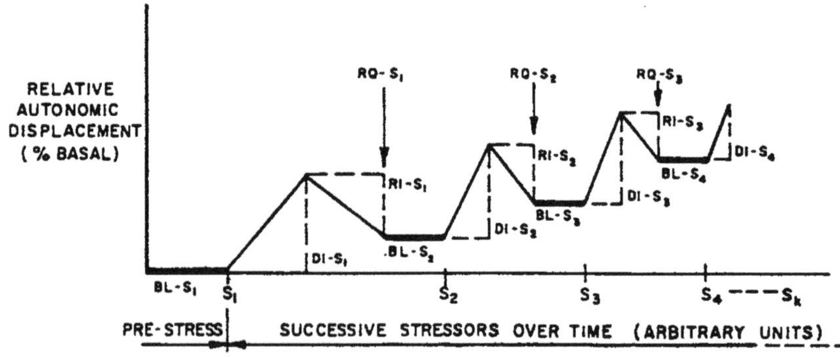

Source: Reference 136, p. 116. Copyright © 1963 by The Free Press, a Division of Macmillan, Inc. Reprinted by permission of Macmillan Publishing Company.

It should be acknowledged at the outset that most of the terms used in Figure 9.3 are similar to those first introduced by G. L. Freeman[38]. Definitions of these terms follow: First, S_1, S_2, S_3, S_4, through S_k refer to the imposition of successive high-SEP stressors, and $BL - S_1$, $BL - S_2$, and so on, refer to the baseline or prestress level of the dependent variable, for example, EDC, at the time the successive stressors were being introduced. Second, $DI - S_1$, $DI - S_2$, and so on, the Displacement Indexes, refer to the percentage change in EDC in this example resulting from S_1, S_2, and so on. $RI - S_1$, $RI - S_2$, and so on, Recovery Indexes, refer to percentage poststress recovery from S_1, S_2, and so on, and $RQ - S_1$, $RQ - S_2$, and so on. Recovery Quotients refer to the ratios of $RI - S_1$ to $DI - S_1$, $RI - S_2$ to $DI - S_2$, and so on (calculated in percentages) following the imposition of S_1, S_2, and so on.

Thus, the stair-stepping model involves the imposition of a series of stressors of varying degrees of SEP, preferably under controlled conditions, such as those found in a laboratory setting. Examples of the type of stress induction procedures for introducing a series of stressors would be a paced motor task or a timed conflict discrimination task. The basic assumption underpinning the stair-stepping hypothesis is that the components of POSR to one stressor are quite different from one individual to another, particularly in terms of the degree of recovery from the accumulative POSR resulting from the imposition of successive high-SEP stressors. Accordingly, the individual differences of interest are the variances in the relative recovery to baseline level as the successive stressors are introduced. The most important operational measure of recovery following exposure to a given stressor is the RQ (Recovery Quotient), calculated from the ratio of the RI (Recovery Index) to the DI (Displacement Index)[38]. Also individual differences in the slopes (tangents of the angle of inclination) of the

RQ's plotted against sequential stressors over time appeared to be a usefully valid predictive index, positive slope predicting compensation and negative slope predicting decompensation (high to low SCC, respectively) in the high-IED situation of concern.

One study in the literature of submarine stress represents a start at validating the stair-stepping hypothesis[133]. Forty nuclear submariners were exposed to three stress-inducing conditions: a pacing task, a discrimination conflict task, and a maximum breath-holding task. The administrative sequence of the three conditions was randomized. Twenty scores derived from measures of EDC and a measure of hand tremor were the major dependent variables. In addition, there were five criterion measures consisting of peer ratings on five traits: tenseness, likability, emotional stability, motivation, and overall potentiality for submarine duty.

An R-technique factor analysis of the 25 × 25 correlation matrix yielded five factors, of which two were clearly interpretable. Factor I (F_1), labeled Optimal Somato-psychological Adjustment, was defined by high factor loadings by all five criterion trait dimensions and by two variables related to the stair-stepping hypothesis, namely, the DI and an index called the E/I (External/Internal) energy mobilization ratio. The E/I ratio was defined as the ratio of hand tremor to DI (change in EDC to imposed high-IED conditions). Overall, high factor scores on F_1 correlated positively with several independent criteria of submariner effectiveness. Factor II (F_2), on the other hand, was not correlated with submariner adjustment. Nonetheless, F_2 was defined mainly by high negative factor loadings by five EDC measures, suggesting a dimension delineated by low ANS resiliency, by slow reaction time to visual stimuli, and by low grades in submarine school. Based upon the general nature of the high-loading variables, F_2 was labeled "Reduced Excitation Level."

METHODOLOGY FOR THE SIRO PROCEDURE

The SIRO procedure has been very generally described in several places earlier in this book. In Chapter 8, it may be recalled, an example of the use of SIRO was presented in the context of a psychiatrist's need to identify the high-SEP stressors associated with his failure to pass the board certification examination for the third time. Very briefly, SIRO involves Q-sorting stressors according to their SEP as judged by the person conducting the SIRO. Referring back to the *What/How/Why* paradigm discussed earlier in this chapter, SIRO is seen as a procedure that focuses on the *What* of the triad, upon what stressors with what SEP's are present in a particular environment at a specified time. The three phases to the SIRO procedure follow:

Phase I. Stressors are first listed separately on Q-cards by the person conducting the SIRO. Three by five index cards are most frequently used for this purpose.

Phase II. The stressors, each written on a Q-card, are rank ordered or Q-sorted according to their SEP's, with rank "1" stressor(s) judged to have the most intense SEP, rank "2" stressor(s) the next highest SEP, and so on to the lowest SEP stressor(s), rank "n," "n" being the highest rank number.

Phase III. Phase III is called the rank transformation phase. Since rank order distributions seldom approximate equal interval scales, it becomes necessary, or at least advisable, to transform the rank scores for each stressor into standard score form so that the SEP for stressor_1, obtained by an SIRO conducted at time t_1, for example, "obnoxious boss" may be meaningfully compared to the SEP of the same stressor obtained by an SIRO conducted by the same person at time t_2, for instance, a year later. This standard score transformation itself is carried out in three steps. First, the rank position for each stressor is converted to a C.E. (centile equivalent) by the formula, C.E. = $(N - r + 0.5) / N$, where N = the total number of stressors (i.e., the number of Q-cards used in the SIRO) and "r" is the rank order position for the particular stressor undergoing the score transformation. The constant 0.5 is added to the numerator of this equation so that the proportion for the lowest ranked stressor, rank N, can never be zero. The C.E. calculation should be carried out to four significant digits.

The second step in this calculation is to convert the C.E. for each stressor to a normalized standard score called a z-score by means of a readily accessible table of areas under the Normal or Gaussian curve. This is done simply by locating an area in the table (usually four digits) that is approximately equal to the C.E. calculated for each stressor, and then to pinpoint as closely as possible the z-score equivalent of that four-digit number. For example, if C.E. = 0.8413, 0.5000, or 0.1587, the normalized z-score equivalents will be 1.0, 0.0, and -1.0, in the same order. Since the z-score distribution ranges approximately from -3 to $+3$ z-score units, in order to simplify the interpretation of each SEP weighing, it becomes necessary to remove the negative z-scores. This is easily done by the application of a simple formula: $T = 10z + 50$, the resulting score being a much-used standard score called the McCall score or T-score. Thus, the rank order score for each stressor becomes a normalized, area-transformed standard score in a T-score distribution with a mean (M) of fifty and an SD of ten T-score units.

There are several advantages to this T-score conversion. Since the stressors are in equivalent units, the SEP for a given stressor obtained from one SIRO may be compared with the SEP of the same stressor yielded by the same person's SIRO completed at a later time. An example of this strategy has already been mentioned in the case of the SEP scores for the "obnoxious boss" stressor calculated for two SIRO's conducted one year apart. Another strategy this T-score conversion makes possible is the comparison between the SIRO's of two or more different people called upon to adapt to the same IED situation at the same time.

Still a third methodological possibility of the T-score conversion is to combine the between-time SIRO data with the between-person SIRO data in the same study. The goal of this combined study would be to shed some light on the complex question of individual differences in the SEP's of specific stressors for two (or more) individuals exposed to the same high-IED environment for a designated period of time.

Since this chapter was written during the last half of 1990, a timely example of this combined SIRO strategy might be obtained from the hypothetical SIRO's conducted by two soldiers bound for duty in Operation Desert Shield, starting in late summer of 1990. Let us assume that both soldiers had undergone comparable training in desert combat strategies and tactics in the U.S. prior to their departure for the Gulf. Each soldier conducts an SIRO immediately after arrival in the Gulf ($SIRO_1$) and again three months or so later in the desert ($SIRO_2$). Table 9.3 contains a tabulation of the hypothetical ranks changed to T-scores for both SIRO's completed by both soldiers. In the interest of brevity, only five stressors are presented. In reality, one would guess that in an IED situation, such as the one Desert Shield posed, the "N," the number of stressors included in the SIRO's, might well be of the order of twenty, one hundred, or even more.

As stated above, with the ranks converted to T-scores, individual differences between the stressor patterns for soldier "A" and soldier "B" can be examined for each of the five stressors. Thus, on $SIRO_1$, the stressor "separation" was ranked by "B" 25 T-score points higher than the same stressor was ranked by "A." Interestingly, this difference had moderated to eight T-score units when the SIRO's were carried out three months later. However, it is important to note that the SEP of the "separation" stressor for "A" had increased twelve T-score points after three months in the desert while the SEP of the same stressor had decreased five points for "B" during the same exposure to this high-IED environment. This difference in the changes in the SEP of this stressor for the two soldiers could have resulted from some seemingly simple cause(s), such as the frequency of mail delivery from "home" or the "bad" or "good" information contained in that mail. Further, the stressor "isolation" had a twenty-seven T-score point higher SEP for "A" as compared with "B" for $SIRO_1$, but the direction of the difference had reversed when the $SIRO_2$ data were collected. The finding that the SEP of the isolation stressor had decreased significantly after three months deployment in the desert for "A," but, at the same time, had increased significantly for "B" may be an indication that the former had greater SCC for this aspect of this particular high-IED situation than did the latter. On the other hand, "excessive heat" appears to be a high-SEP stressor for both of the soldiers for $SIRO_1$, but it is very much lower for both after three months in the desert, suggesting either a favorable change in the weather or more adequate adaptation to the heat stressor.

The stressor "threat to life and limb," however, is clearly the highest SEP stressor for both "A" and "B" at the beginning as well as after three months into the tour of duty. Finally, with the T-scores for both "A" and "B" in the thirties and low forties for both SIRO's, the stressor "scorpions" would not be expected to contribute substantially to an elevated POSR regardless of the duration of the deployment in the Gulf.

Equation 4.2 is the general formula for calculating the IED (Intensity of

Table 9.3
Hypothetical SIRO Data for Two Desert Shield Soldiers

Stressors	Ranks				Centile Equivalents[d]				z-scores				T-scores			
	A_1[a]	A_2	B_1	B_2	A_1	A_2	B_1	B_2	A_1	A_2	B_1	B_2	A_1	A_2	B_1	B_2
N[b]	10	14	15	18												
excessive heat	1	4	3	7	950	750	833	639	1.65	0.68	0.95	0.36	66	57	60	54
threat to life and limb	1	1	2	1	950	964	900	972	1.65	1.80	1.29	1.91	66	68	63	69
separation	8	5	1	6	250	678	966	694	-0.67	0.46	1.83	0.51	43	55	68	63
isolation	2	9	14	9	850	392	100	528	1.40	-0.27	-1.28	0.07	64	47	37	51
scorpions	9	14	12	16	150	075	230	139	-1.30	-1.40	-0.74	-1.08	37	36	43	39
I.E.D.[c]													276	263	271	276

[a] A_1, A_2, B_1, B_2 -- are the data for soldiers A and B for $SIRO_1$ and $SIRO_2$ respectively.
[b] N -- Number of stressors in the Q-sort distribution; five stressors were selcted from these distributions for this scoring demonstration.
[c] I.E.D. -- Intensity of Environmental Demands
[d] Decimals are omitted.

Environmental Demands). A more detailed formulation for calculating IED with the stressors in the required T-score form is as follows:

$$IED = n_1T_1 + n_2T_2 + \dots . n_kT_k,$$

where, n_1, n_2. . . . n_k are the number of stressors in the rank 1, rank 2, and so on to the kth rank position, each multiplied by the T-score for the stressor(s) with that rank. Obviously, if there is only one stressor in each rank position (i.e., $n_1 = n_2 = n_k$), IED can be calculated by simply summing all of the T-scores in the SIRO distribution. It should be noted that in Table 9.3 the IED's for both "A" and "B" calculated from the $SIRO_1$ data are roughly the same as the IED's yielded by $SIRO_2$, conducted three months later. It might be inferred from these IED levels that the POSR associated with these desert stressors apparently were relatively constant for both of these legendary soldiers after three months' battle-preparation training.

Although the SIRO data in Table 9.3 are hypothetical, nonetheless, the score conversion methodology and the several interpretive statements regarding the score patterns are presented here as instructional information to be used as guidelines for anyone, lay or professional, contemplating the application of the SIRO procedure to real-life situations.

This chapter ends as it began, with a cogent admonition for the scientist by my colleague and mentor, Dr. Walter Miles. Some years before his death when he was in his eighties, Dr. Miles said to me, "I have only one regret—I won't be able to conduct my own autopsy. Think what I might find out about myself! The problem is we do not have the appropriate methodology." "You see," Dr. Miles went on, "*How* we analyze our data is just as important as *What* data we analyze." Hence this chapter.

10

Looking Forward by Looking Backward: The ABC Solution

In the preface to this text, after a brief discussion of the volume and fragmentation of the stress literature to date, the question was asked, "So, why add another book on the subject of stress to this literary clutter?" The justification for writing the ten chapters that followed that question was based on the assumption that the ABC model of stress, presented in Figure 3.1, would provide new insights regarding some of the contemporary social issues related to the topic. A second, more specific assumption is made at this time, namely, that by looking backward in this text at the manner in which the basic concepts associated with the ABC model were developed and applied, it is possible to look forward for explanations and perhaps some mitigating factors for some of the most critical social, geopolitical, and cultural problems of our time.

Throughout the history of psychology, a dilemma in theorizing about the causes of human behavior at a given time and in a circumscribed environment has persisted[64, 70]. This dilemma is: should the emphasis be *historical* (that is, based on the premise that present behavior results from a past developmental series of maturation and learning processes) or *ahistorical* (that is, based on the premise that the causes of present behavior are to be found in the environmental and phenomenological "field" of the person at the time the behavior occurs). The former set of causal assumptions are espoused by the Freudian psychoanalytic school and the latter by the Lewinian field theoretical school[64, 70]. Fortunately, the ABC model is eclectic in that it represents an attempt to understand stress-related behavior in terms of both historical and ahistorical influences.

EDUCATIONAL DEFICIENCIES AND THE ABC MODEL

In the search for applications of the ABC model to contemporary problems, a timely place to start seemed to be the long-standing issue of deficiencies in the educational systems in the U.S. Soon after his inauguration, President Bush stated that he wanted to be remembered as the educational president, a statement that attests to the high priority of the educational issue in modern times. Consistent with the president's statement, the summary report from the governors' conference on education called by President Bush indicated that the major educational deficiencies had been identified. Insufficient funding, the poor quality of teachers, and minority segregation and discrimination were some of the problem areas mentioned in the conference report. Those deficiencies were based upon such normative data as below average SAT (Scholastic Aptitude Test) scores, a 20 to 40 percent high school dropout rate, reading skills of high school graduates at the sixth-grade level, and so on. Concomitant symptoms of these substandard performance indicators were also discussed at the conference, symptoms such as drug abuse, teenage pregnancy, truancy, violence, delinquency, AIDS, and criminal behavior.

In general, the outcome of the conference was substantive in terms of long-range planning (higher taxes to increase teachers' salaries, for example) but was lacking in the sense of developing even a dim outline of the most appropriate methods or approaches for mitigating or removing the causes of these signs and symptoms.

What recommendations for addressing these deficiencies can be inferred from the ABC model (Figure 3.1) and the concepts generated by the model? Before attempting to answer this question, it is necessary to make two additional assumptions, emphasizing both historical and ahistorical factors. These are: (1) that the overt signs and symptoms, substandard performance, truancy, dropout rate, drug abuse, and violence, for example, have a fundamental cause or at least a concomitant, namely *chronically elevated POSR*, and (2) the immediate causes of this high POSR level and the resulting maladaptive indicators as well as suggestions for their alleviation or removal may be found in the ABC model and the three equations emanating from that model. These three equations are reiterated here for convenience (see original equations for definition of symbols).

Equation 4.1

$$POSR_{jr} = K_j \frac{IED_r}{AR_j}$$

Equation 4.2

$$IED_{jr} = SEP_{Stressor\ I} + SEP_{Stressor\ II} + \ldots SEP_{Stressor\ k}$$

Equation 4.3

POSR = (f) A. Effect of "mods"
B. IED/AR ratio
C. Expectancy of Outcome Ratio, $RF^{\pm}/Pu^{\pm}$
D. Valence of Goals or Outcomes
E. Clarity of PRC's and ARC's

One cause of the deficiencies in the educational system is related to the developmental histories of the students themselves. Turning to Phase I of the ABC model (Figure 3.1), it is seen that childhood and early adolescence are the developmental periods during which the NPP's are formed through the processes of maturation and learning. Assuming that primary needs tend to be satisfied in most cases, the prepotency of secondary needs, such as affiliation, self-esteem, and achievement, depends upon two factors occurring in Phases II and III of the ABC model. These two factors are: first, whether the energy mobilized by a particular need becomes repeatedly (habitually) channeled by *effective* PRC's and ARC's so as to maximize the expectancy of a high OR and, second, which of the classes of stressors typical of this developmental time frame becomes persistent and takes on high-SEP (*see* Table 5.1). Occurring during the first ten to twelve years of a normal life-span, these two kinds of stress-related processes directly affect the attitude and value profiles underpinning many students' lifelong life-styles or personalities. Should the patterns of high-SEP stressors encountered during the early developmental time frame persist throughout the educational years, the IED and the correlated POSR will likewise be sustained at high levels, the result being significantly reduced overall SCC. Further, dropout, drug abuse, and delinquency are also some of the likely behavioral concomitants of sustained, high-level POSR. Thus, the following educational principles emerge from the above discussion of these selected concepts derived from the ABC model.

Educational Principle I

It is implied from the above discussion that chronically elevated POSR during crucial developmental periods tend to generate socially unacceptable value systems and asocial or antisocial, negative (avoidance) attitudes. One common example of such attitudes and values frequently found in students is a new addition to the psychiatric nomenclature, schoolphobia. Equation 4.1 presented above suggests that POSR may be prevented from becoming excessive by controlling the IED levels during these educational years. Equation 4.2, in turn, implies that the level of IED may be controlled, or at least monitored, by conducting periodic stressor audits or SIRO procedures, particularly during the late adolescent and early adult period. SIRO data collected during this time span would serve to identify the high-SEP stressors prevailing during each developmental stage (see Table 5.1). Having delineated the high-SEP stressors typical of each developmental interval, the MEL or MEL's are determined and the most appropriate IVP's for the localized stressors can then be selected and applied (see Tables 8.1 and 8.2).

An example of the application of this educational principle follows: Let us consider a fourth grader who, with a long-standing history of truancy and failing grades, discloses during a SIRO conducted by the student assisted by the school counselor that, because of a minor speech impairment, she/he becomes very fearful when asked to speak or read aloud in class. In the language of "ABC," the POSR likely to occur in this situation most probably results from "anticipated blockage of goal-directed behavior," or, stated differently, the high IED caused by the group's demand "to speak!" produces intense POSR, which, in turn, tend to produce avoidance behavior (truancy) and negative attitudes, both sustained by repeated negative reinforcement (RF−). Stated more simply, the student feels better (RF−) as a result of carrying out the only PRC she/he knows, "stay away from the group."[11, 93]

To reiterate, based upon the assumption that many of the maladaptive symptoms of students described above result from sustained high-level POSR, Educational Principle I states that POSR can be controlled by reducing the IED level expressed as the numerator of the IED/AR ratio in Equation 4.1. This strategy should reduce the classroom avoidance motivation of the fourth grader in the above example.

To continue the example, having identified the high-SEP stressors by SIRO, (examples of stressors for the fourth grader might be "classmates' impatience when I stutter," "my teacher's irritability," or "classmates avoid me"), the most effective IVP's for reducing the IED for the student should be applied. Thus, based upon these SIRO data, the most appropriate MEL seems to be the group level (*see* Table 8.1). The ABC model suggests that the IED and, hence, the POSR of the student can be reduced in the following ways: (1) by removing as many of the high-SEP stressors associated with the classroom situation as possible, an insensitive peer who laughs at her/him when speech hesitancies occur, for example and (2) by reducing the SEP of selected stressors functioning as a significant part of the student's perception of the group as a whole. An example might be to educate the student's teachers (who, in turn, educate their students) about the concept of "social feedback." That is, clearly describe the unpleasant effect that the student experiences upon noticing his or her classmates' adverse reactions to the stress-inducing attempts to speak while in the group.

Overall, the recommendations from the ABC model for reducing the IED level for the student in our example is to remove as many high-SEP stressors as possible from the educational situation and to increase his/her expectancy that the OR (that is, more $RF^{\pm}$ than $Pu^{\pm}$) will be maximized within the classroom and other educational situations. As a result, the severity of the student's school-phobic symptoms should also be significantly reduced.

Educational Principle II

Still based on Equation 4.1, the intensity of POSR can be controlled not only by reducing the IED, but also by increasing the AR of the students. By increasing the AR of the child or adolescent in the educational context, the overall SCC of the students to adjust to stressors beyond the classroom will also be enhanced. Throughout the two early developmental periods (*see* Figure 3.1), both AR and SCC can be increased for the developing person by assisting him/her in selecting and applying effective PRC's and ARC's for the specific high-SEP stressors identified by the periodic stressor audits or SIRO's recommended by Educational Principle I. As indicated in Equation 4.3, it follows that the more clearly defined and the more accessible effective PRC's and ARC's are for a given set of stressors confronted during childhood and adolescence, the less intense the POSR caused by these stressors will be and the more adequate the SCC of the developing person will be during these and later developmental periods (*see* Table 5.1).

The example of the fourth grader with a speech handicap described above also serves to illustrate Principle II. Thus, it is possible for a qualified speech therapist, by teaching the student several contingencies (relaxation and word-forming techniques, for instance) for producing articulate speech in a classroom setting, to reduce significantly the POSR intensity level, and, overall, to enhance the SCC of this particular student for this specific set of environmental stressors. Coupled with the effects of IED reduction by means of Principle I, the establishment of effective PRC's and ARC's will reduce the tendency to develop negative attitudes and socially unacceptable values, often part of the school-phobic syndrome. Complementing the effects of the application of Principle I, the application of Education Principle II will also increase the student's expectancy that his her school-related activities will result in maximizing the OR, by increasing the likelihood of more $RF^{\pm}$ than $Pu^{\pm}$. Finally, it becomes more likely that she/he will develop sustained lifelong motivation "to learn" and to achieve meaningful educational goals. These stable motives, attitudes, and values, if developed early, should similarly increase his/her SCC for some of the high-SEP stressors of adulthood.

Possible generalizations from this one example of the application of Educational Principles I and II to other aspects of the educational process are numerous and varied (for example, the development of effective study habits as well as important communication and other social skills). It would appear that the same general principles inferred from the ABC model would apply not only to educational settings, but also to business and a variety of community settings as well.

CREATIVITY AND THE ABC MODEL OF STRESS

To search for a definition of a reified term, such as "creativity," is to look for a black cat in a dark room with all of the shades drawn. Therefore, when the word "creativity" is used in the following discussion, it will be referring to creative behavior or creative activity. In this sense then, creative behavior can be operationally defined as the process(es) by means of which an old problem is solved in new ways. Thomas A. Edison noticed that artificial light had been produced for centuries by burning combustible material in the presence of air, but when the combustible material was gone, so was the light. He reasoned further that it was the oxygen component of air that supported the combustion; therefore, if some sort of material could be heated in a relatively air-free chamber, light would be produced by the heated material, later on to be called a filament. Moreover, he reasoned that if this filament were heated in a vacuum, since very little oxygen would be present, it would have its combustion time greatly extended, so the incandescent light was created.

There are two broad aspects of creative activity that have interested psychologists since World War II: first, the personality trait patterns characterizing creative persons as compared to noncreative persons, and second, the kind of environmental circumstances that are conducive to creative behavior in general[76]. As we shall see, the ABC model contains suggestions mainly for the second of these two aspects of creativity, that is, processes related to initiating, sustaining, and reinforcing creative ideation and behavior[7].

L. L. Thurstone, more than four decades ago, conducted several comprehensive studies of both of these aspects of creativity[120]. The findings from this series of studies suggested that the personality of creative persons is characterized by both intellectual and temperamental traits. Academic intelligence as measured by IQ tests is only slightly correlated with creative productivity. However, something like the trait of "open-mindedness" and a noncritical attitude toward novel ideas are typically found in creative persons. Creative ideation and the psychoimagery by which a developmental plan of action for these ideas seem to occur not when the potential creator is concentrating on the problem at hand, but instead when she/he is in a relaxed (nontense) state with widely dispersed or nonfocused attention. An ancient, yet appropriate example of this creative mood state or mind set might be the story of the Athenian, Archimedes, who discovered his all-important buoyancy principle (critical for the functioning of a submarine, by the way) while sitting quietly in an overflowing bathtub. "Eureka! I have found it" was his excited announcement of his discovery.

Is the ability to carry out creative activity the result of biological predispositions or the effects of learning? As with functional intelligence as measured by IQ tests, creative ability seems to be the result of the interaction of both nature and nurture. Particularly in the arts, the biogenetic predispositional factors appear to contribute disproportionately more to creativity than, for example, general intelligence. An anecdote about one of the most creative musical geniuses, Wolfgang Amadeus Mozart, makes the point very well. It seems a 50-year-old musician, upon meeting Mozart in a Vienna courtyard, asked, "Mr. Mozart, how do you go about composing a piece of music?" Mozart, looking somewhat distainfully at the man, replied, "You are too young to compose music." "But sir, you composed a delightful little sonata for piano and violin when you were only five." "This is true," Mozart said in his characteristic haughty style, "but," he added, "I didn't have to ask anyone how to go about doing it."

A ten-year series of R-technique factor analytical studies of creativity was reported by Dr. J. P. Guilford in 1959[47]. These studies produced the so-called SI (structure-of-intellect) model. SI came to be accepted as the most comprehensive frame of reference for the study of creativity. The most important bipolar factors produced by an R-technique factor analysis of a battery of tests of creativity and included in the SI model was labeled the divergent/convergent dimension. Convergent thinking, required to respond effectively to multiple-choice tests, consists of obtaining a *single* solution based upon a set of given facts. Divergent thinking, on the other hand, is much less constrained by specified facts, thus resulting in the possibility of arriving at a diversity of solutions to the same problem. Most of the available evidence argues that persons whose problem-solving style tends to be more divergent than convergent, in general, would be expected to produce more creative end products or results.

Some of the implications of the ABC model suggest several principles by which creative activity of selected persons may be maximized. For this purpose, the most useful recommendations from the ABC model involve the computer-age principles derived from a servomechanistic paradigm. Servomechanistic systems involve three elements: input, mediation processes, and output. The analogy to the ABC model—antecedents (A), behavioral contingency(ies) (B), and consequences (C)—is obvious. Insofar as creativity is concerned, there are two general propositions that flow from the servocontrol notion: first, creative behavior will be maximized to the degree that *feedforward* processes are explicit, feasible, and lead to adequate reinforcement; and, second, the greater the degree to which positive feedbackward exceeds negative feedbackward as reinforcement for presumed creative activity, the greater will be the motivation to initiate and sustain novel, imaginative behavior.

As discussed earlier in the section describing the ABC model, the most appropriate example of feedforward processes is a typical computer program consisting of an algorithm, a recipe or a set of instructions by which input information is transformed into a desired outcome, event, or end state. PRC's and ARC's in the ABC model are feedforward processes (the "B" in the model) that, in the case of creativity, refer to the goal-directed behavior, or the reinforcement contingencies, most effective for solving an old problem in a new way.

Also discussed earlier are the feedbackward processes, a very important aspect of the ABC model. In the language of computers, feedbackward processes refer to the effects of output "C" working backwards in such a manner as to affect the input "A," the antecedents or activators in Figure 3.1. In other words, insofar as creativity is concerned, the consequences or outcomes of a presumed creative contingency or set of contingencies would be expected to feedback upon the input or antecedents for other similar activity. In general, feedback is negative if it tends to suppress further creative behavior and positive if it tends to enhance it.

To reiterate, the ABC model indicates that when immediately perceived or anticipated blockage of goal-directed behavior occurs, strong emotional reactivity called stress or, more appropriately, POSR, is the consequence. As previously discussed, however, some level of POSR seems to be beneficial, even necessary. It may be further recalled that Hans Selye labeled this beneficial POSR "eustress," meaning, literally, good stress[105]. In fact, moderate POSR may result in the potential creator's sorting through a variety of possible RC's for achieving the desired creative end product(s) or outcomes. An excellent example of this persistent trial-and-error effort to find the most appropriate RC or RC's for a critical problem is to be found in the research activity of Dr. Paul Ehrlich, the renowned physician, bacteriologist, and chemist. Around the turn of the century, the incidence of the venereal disease syphilis was increasing at an astronomical rate. Dr. Ehrlich and his colleagues, desperately searching for a bactericide for the syphilis spirochete, discovered the drug salvarsan, which turned out to be the first successful cure for the dreaded disease. Salvarsan came to be called "606" after the fact that 606 different compounds had been tested before salvarsan was finally identified.

In sum, the ABC model suggests several prescriptions for maximizing creative behavior, suggestions derived mainly from the feedback concept, which, as indicated above, is an integral part of the model. Specifically, these prescriptions involve three kinds of processes: those techniques that enhance feedforward processes, those that maximize positive feedback, and those that minimize negative feedback.

Enhancing Feedforward Processes

The ABC model suggests several major strategies by which feedforward processes can be enhanced. In the first place, antecedents or activators ("A" in ABC) initiate the energy channelization processes by which motivational vectors take on directional properties. "A" can be any kind of stimulus situation that attracts the creative person and functions as an impetus or activator for creative activity. "A" might be an environmental irritant, a stressor that generates energy mobilization, and the channeling of a motivational vector toward solving a challenging problem. In some instances, "A" provokes the "what if" type of question: What if I change this, or what if I tried this or that, and so forth. For example, in modern times, there is a very critical, almost frantic, need to find an effective biochemical or pharmacological agent that cures, or at least retards, the lethal course of the disease AIDS. Virologists, microbiologists, pharmacologists, and other specialists, armed with the information that the etiological basis for AIDS is the HIV (human immuno-virus), are channeling great amounts of resources in a number of directions in an attempt to find an antidote for that specific pathogen. In the case of AIDS, the "A," the initiating force in the feedforward process, is strong and compelling—in one specific instance, to prevent AIDS-inflicted genocide of certain cultural groups in North Africa.

In other situations, evoking the motivational vector "to create" (to solve a specific problem in a new way) is not so compelling. Consider, for example, the kinds of ideas, new products, and new problem-solving approaches to old problems that might emerge if teachers and parents, sensing creative potential in a developing youngster, would initiate creative motivation (the "A" in ABC) by raising challenging questions and encouraging a variety of responses to such crucial social problems as illiteracy, drug abuse, and poverty. If the antecedent conditions are sufficiently compelling and, as we shall see below, the feedforward processes are sustained by appropriate reinforcers, there may be no practical limit to the creative production of a selected segment of the population.

A second strategy by which feedforward processes may be maximized is to provide access to an array of different PRC's for accomplishing a clearly specified creative goal. In addition to providing new PRC's, feedforward processes are made more efficient by clarification of existing PRC's and ARC's. For instance, returning to the urgent problem of finding an AIDS cure, it is known that the T-lymphotropic virus type-III (HTLV-III) attacks the immune system by invading the bodies of certain white blood cells called T-cell lymphocytes. Within these cells, the virus is apparently impervious to experimental drugs of any kind. Unfortunately, drugs sufficiently potent to destroy the HTLV-III also destroy the white blood cell at the same time. Accordingly, a possible PRC might be to search for an explanation of the process by which the HTLV-III penetrates the lymphocytes in the first place. Were this mechanism thoroughly understood, then a drug or other substance might be developed to prevent the invasion of the virus into the blood system, thus leaving the AIDS virus more vulnerable to virucidal agents of several types. Should this happen, a modified PRC will have been developed to enhance the feedforward process toward the achievement of the goal of preventing AIDS.

A third approach to enhance feedforward processes is to develop means by which barriers to creative RC's are removed or made more permeable or circumventable. The reduction of the perceived imperviousness of the barriers to creative contingencies has two important consequences: reduction of the POSR caused by anticipating blockage of the creative contingency and that of increasing the expectancy that the OR will be maximized (*see* Equation 4.3). As Table 5.1 indicates, there are several classes of barriers or stressors that may impede or block creative contingencies. These blockages can be political, economic, physical, or sociocultural in nature. As suggested in the discussion of IVP's for excessive POSR in Chapter 8, having identified the high-SEP stressors that are blocking or impeding the creative activity, the IVP's that are selected depend to a considerable degree upon the nature of the stressor(s) (Table 5.1). Only in rare instances are physical stressors, such as excessive heat, cold, and noise, of any great concern for impeding creative behavior, but sociocultural and attitudinal stressors may take on high-SEP properties when creative behavior related to social or geopolitical issues is involved. For example, Irving Janis's concept of "groupthink" functioned as a harsh barrier to the development of creative recommendations while President Kennedy's Bay of Pigs campaign was being planned in 1961[58]. With the exception of Secretary Schlesinger, all of the members of the president's cabinet were reluctant to show openly nonconforming attitudes to the "apparent" consensus decision to implement the ill-planned, militarily indefensible mission. "Don't bother the president with new [translation, creative] ideas; the president has already made up his mind," Robert Kennedy, then attorney general, is said to have stated. "Be intelligent—think as I do" is a similar dictum often implied in modern social intercourse. Thus, the opportunity to propose alternative approaches (that is, new PRC's and ARC's) to accomplish the goal of ousting Castro was blocked by the expectancy of a very low OR—that is, a higher likelihood of $Pu^{\pm}$ than of $RF^{\pm}$ (*see* Equation 4.3). Blockage of creative contingencies by groupthink, which may be described as a "fear-of-nonconforming" stressor, is most clearly demonstrable when social, religious, and political issues are at stake. Note, for instance, the threatened excommunication of Governor Mario Cuomo from the Roman Catholic church for openly expressing his right-to-choose bias in the politically explosive abortion issue.

Once sociocultural or other barriers (stressors) to creative feedforward processes are identified by SIRO, appropriate IVP(s) should be applied either to remove the barriers, or make them more permeable or circumventable[45, 46]. For example, in the case of the groupthink stressor and its interference with the efficiency of group problem solving, a useful IVP to apply is some standardized procedure, such as the Delphi technique[73]. Briefly, the Delphi technique, a group problem-solving approach typically used to solve very complex problems, requires each member of a designated problem-solving group to respond to a series of questionnaires focused on various aspects of the issue at hand. Anonymous answers to these questionnaire items are studied by all members of the group and are integrated later into a single solution, or, in some cases, listed in a series of prioritized solutions. The groupthink effect is avoided by this technique, since there are no barriers to an individual's anonymous creative ideas being submitted as questionnaire responses.

Finally, feedforward processes by which creative contingencies will be reinforced are obviously affected by the nature of the consequences following the creative activity, the "C" in the ABC model. Appropriate manipulation of any or all of the elements in Equation 4.3 will improve the effectiveness of the feedforward processes related to a variety of creative contingencies. Accordingly, the efficacy of feedforward processes of this kind is favorably affected by (1) exploiting moderator variables, such as unique aptitudes, specialized education or experience, and so on; (2) reducing the POSR of the person or persons involved by mitigating the intensity of IED (e.g., reducing the conformity pressure in a group problem-solving situation); (3) increasing the positive valence of the creative goal(s) or outcome(s) and/or reducing their negative valence; (4) increasing the AR of the creative person(s), by specialized training, for example; (5) sustaining a high expectancy that creative contingencies will result in a high OR; and, finally, (6) maximizing positive feedback as reinforcement for developing and implementing creative contingencies. The effects of feedbackward processes for maintaining creative contingencies will be discussed next.

Feedbackward Processes and Creativity

It is well to reiterate a general principle describing the relationship between creativity and feedbackward processes. In general, the greater the degree to which positive feedback exceeds negative feedback as reinforcement for creative activity, the greater the motivation will be to initiate new and eliminate ineffective ongoing contingencies aimed at the same goal or outcome.

There are two types of feedback: extrinsic and intrinsic[90]. Extrinsic feedback consists of external or palpable consequences (in the case of creativity, the completion of a series of creative contingencies resulting in a "new" product or outcome). An example of positive extrinsic feedback might be the awarding of a large monetary award (the Nobel Prize, for example) for a prestigious scientific discovery or invention. On the other hand, an example of negative extrinsic feedback would be a doctoral candidate whose dissertation chairman candidly states that her/his dissertation proposal is unacceptable because it lacks originality. In contrast to extrinsic feedback, intrinsic feedback involves the creator's own internal self-evaluation of the consequences of his/her own creative behavior. For instance, an artist's experience of satisfaction or sense of accomplishment with a painting or musical composition would function as positive intrinsic feedback for continuing the creative activity. Another example of positive intrinsic feedback might be the Yankee slugger Mickey Mantle's description of his experience upon hitting a home run, "it just feels right." Examples of negative intrinsic feedback are plentiful. One such example might be the negative emotional experience (−AC), actually the POSR, that a student endures upon completing a final "exam" and realizing that most of the test questions had been taken from subject matter not included in the student's "exam" preparation.

Overall, the rather straightforward principle emerges: negative feedbackward processes, both extrinsic and intrinsic, as consequences for creative activity function as Pu−, thus tending to suppress creativity. Conversely, positive feedback, similarly extrinsic or intrinsic, functions as RF+, resulting in enhanced creative behavior.

In sum, consistent with the overlying theme of the ABC model and of the text as a whole, any manipulation, procedure, or process by means of which reinforcement contingencies, creative or otherwise, are made more efficient serves to reduce POSR and, at the same time, increase the expectancy of a high OR. The end result is a significant improvement in individual SCC, often resulting in enhanced creative production.

LEADERSHIP BEHAVIOR AND THE ABC MODEL

If the number of papers published and the number of symposia conducted on some one or another aspect of the topic of leadership are the criteria, the subject of leadership has gained tremendous popularity within both the lay and scientific communities since World War II[35, 122]. The majority of these endeavors have tended to reify the concept "leadership" as an entity to be sought out and found for study and observation. It has been emphasized throughout this book that the proper subject matter of science has as its referent a body of inferences originating from sensory, palpable data. Accordingly, leadership activity or leadership behavior, rather than the entity "leadership" is the focus of this segment of this chapter.

Inferred from interpersonal activity within a circumscribed group, LB (leadership behavior) consists of whatever one or more persons do within that group that produces a significant change (preferably enhancement) in the motivation and performance of the group members toward achieving group-relevant goals. The operative clause of this definition is "whatever one or more persons do." It follows therefore, that the focus of the study of leadership behavior should be upon the mechanisms or processes involved in the strengthening of the motivation, quality of member interpersonal relationships, and the efficacy of their performance in a group setting. More specifically, modern leadership theory suggests that researchers on the topic focus on five general subject matter areas: (1) the personality characteristics of the person or persons in leadership positions within a given group; (2) the processes or mechanisms inherent in effective LB itself; (3) the roles, the communication networks, and other interpersonal relationships of the group members; (4) the purpose(s), goals, and the developmental history of the group; and (5) the environmental context in which the group functions.

Before we suggest possible applications of the ABC model to these subject matter areas related to LB, however, one pervasive theoretical issue should be addressed, namely, the nature/nurture controversy[35, 55]. The effectiveness of LB has historically been considered a function of certain personality trait patterns of the person occupying leadership positions in a specific group. At present, the pendulum of leadership theory appears to have swung from the "nature" notion that leaders are born (that is, that LB results from biogenetic predispositions) toward the nurture notion that leaders are made (that is, that LB results from maturation and learning). Generally speaking, the recent empirical literature addressing this theoretical dilemma argues strongly that such trait patterns as intelligence, aggressiveness, body build, and the like are not consistently found in persons exhibiting effective LB and are absent in nonleaders. Rather, the nature of LB as well as its predictability from one group to another result from the *interaction* of "nature and nurture", that is, the interaction between selected personality traits of the potential leader; his or her learned leadership skills; and the history, objectives, structure, and environmental context of the particular group of interest.

Thus, assuming that the potential leader finds herself or himself in a favorable power position within a given group, certain recommendations for effective LB are suggested by the ABC model and the equations emanating from it. These are:

1. The goal(s) or purpose(s) of the group's existence must be clearly stated, preferably written, and explained fully.
2. The valence or significance of the group goals and expected outcomes or end products should be convincingly explained.
3. An array of clearly delineated contingencies (PRC's and ARC's), appropriate for achieving the group goals, should be manifestly spelled out for the group members, and, in some cases, prioritized.

4. Every possible effort should be made to maximize the expectancy of each group member's realizing a high OR ($RF^{\pm}/Pu^{\pm}$) as a result of his/her group participation.
5. Finally, provide assurance that intragroup communication channels will be kept open and that periodic feedback pertaining to each member's progress toward goal accomplishment will be forthcoming.

The CCNW (Co-contingency Network) Theory of Leadership

The impetus for the CCNW theory of leadership had its origin in a basic survival mechanism in the field of biology and physical chemistry. Vital functions of higher animals, including humans, are sustained not only by a number of homeostatic mechanisms, but also by an important physical and chemical process called agglutination, literally "a gluing together" of blood cells or bacteria into clots or clusters functioning as a unit. These groupings of biological matter are controlled by the laws of physics and chemistry. These clots and clusters serve a critical survival function by preventing hemorrhage and as counteractants for disease and other pathological processes.

Although the analogy is only approximate, clusters of people called groups consist of persons with some kind of interperson affinity and functioning more or less in concert to accomplish meaningful group objectives. Also, like the nucleus of a blood cell, there is generally within the group a person or persons who somehow influence the activity of the other group members in such a way as to affect the functional and structural characteristics of the group as well as the productivity and survivability of its members.

The CCNW theory of LB is based upon the notion that once the goals of a group are clearly known and understood by the group members and the contingencies by which these goals are to be achieved have been clearly spelled out, a unique class of interpersonal processes can be initiated and, if properly reinforced, can be sustained within the group. Reciprocally reinforcing processes between and among group members develop from the incorporation of individual motivational vectors (see Figures 2.1 and 3.1). These coalesced vectors, first as dyads, then triads, quadrads, and so on, are called CC's (co-contingencies) for shared goals. In turn, concatenations of CC's, again mutually reinforcing, become CCNW's functioning as coalesced motivational vectors within the circumscribed group.

A possibly frivolous example of CC formation and the transition to CCNW's implied by the CCNW theory may be found in Mark Twain's *Huckleberry Finn* when Aunt Polly persuaded a reluctant "Huck" to whitewash her badly peeling picket fence. First, Huck, the PL (potential leader) sets out to enhance the positive valence of the whitewashing task. To do this, the PL pointed out to his friend (let us call him $chum_1$) how good Aunt Polly would feel to have her fence whitewashed; moreover, $chum_1$ was reminded how well known Aunt Polly's homemade fruit pies were in the neighborhood. The next step in the PL's developing leadership strategy was to produce for himself and $chum_1$ the brushes, buckets, and limewater necessary to start the task. Then, $chum_2$ appears, notes $chum_1$ busily whitewashing, and, with some exhortation from the PL, pitches in to help $chum_1$. Thus, the motivational vectors of $chum_1$ and $chum_2$ have become conjoined as one vector, thus forming CC_1 (co-contingency number one). The PL then reinforces the coordinated CC_1 activity with some contemporary slang, such as "nice going" or "bully for you." Whereupon PL temporarily withdraws to recruit $chum_3$ and $chum_4$ and, following some discussion about the goals of the project, CC_2 is formed. The PL uses the same sequence of actions to recruit $chum_5$, $chum_6$, and so on.

Finally, the coalescence of the CC's now functioning within the group results in the formation of a CCNW, a cohesive subgroup focused on a common goal, namely, to get the fence whitewashed. In turn, the reciprocal, interpersonal reinforcement within the CCNW(s) now begins to function in such a way as to sustain the group motivation until the goal or outcome (a whitewashed fence) has been achieved by the co-contingent effort of the total group.

Using a literary classic to demonstrate certain principles of leadership style implied by the CCNW theory of LB suggests a general prescription for implementation of the requirements of the theory. This prescription consists of an expansion of a series of steps or phases similar to those used by "Huck" to get Aunt Polly's fence whitewashed. These principles, stated in the language of the ABC model, consist of a series of eight phases, as follows:

1. *Situation description phase*. The structure, the goals, and the purpose(s) of the group are clearly explained and discussed.
2. *Valence enhancement phase*. The significance of the accomplishment of the group goals by coordinated group member activity is stated in objective terms.
3. *Contingency clarification phase*. A specific delineation of an array of contingencies available to group members for achieving high-valent group and individual goals is presented. Prioritization of these contingencies may be possible in some instances. Further, cinematic demonstrations or *in vivo* modeling may be useful in this context.
4. *Expectancy enhancement phase*. Increase the subjective probability that collaborative effort of the group members will result in a maximum OR ($RF^{\pm}/Pu^{\pm}$). Minimize the expectancy of encountering insurmountable high-SEP stressors.
5. *CC (co-contingency) clarification phase*. Emphasize and, in some instances, demonstrate that shared goal-directed activity (CC's) of group members is generally more mutually satisfying and effective than individual member activity. Give examples of CC's as the most effective means for achieving group goals.
6. *Co-contingency reinforcement phase*. Group members in the process of

carrying out CC's are reinforced by pointing to objective evidence of progress toward shared goals.

7. *CCNW (co-contingency network) formation phase*. Combinations of CC's are reinforced, thereby forming CCNW's. It might be advisable to demonstrate that individual motivational vectors coalesce into CC's, which, in turn, combine to form CCNW's, the result being high member satisfaction and enhanced quality and quantity of group performance.
8. *CCNW (co-contingency network) reinforcement phase*. The CC's, now combined into CCNW's, are similarly reinforced by again noting progress toward the achievement of the high-valent group goals.

Since substantive empirical validation is lacking, the CCNW theory of LB stands as a series of working hypotheses, no more, no less. In science, hypotheses function as educated guesses requiring testing and factual support. It may be recalled that the word "heuristic" has been used frequently throughout the ABC text. In the case of the CCNW theory, investigative opportunities abound. For example, a three-group, controlled experiment with a before and after leadership skills training feature could easily be designed. The objective of such an experiment would be to assess the relative efficacy of the CCNW approach as a pedagogical program for leadership skills training. The experimental setting could be some kind of group task, such as the one of erecting a tent used in the prison guard experiment described earlier (reference number 132). Designated PL's in two of the three randomly selected groups of ten or so would have been thoroughly trained in one of two leadership styles: authoritarian or instrumental style[35, 55] or the CCNW, eight-phase style described above. The third PL would receive some general instructions, such as "see how quickly you can get this ten-person group to erect this tent." The operational definitions of the experimental or dependent variables could be: time to complete the task or the quality of the end result as indicated by the approximation to the vertical of the tent, the stability of the tent provided by the placement of the stakes, and so on. An ANOVA (analysis of variance; *see* Glossary) would definitely shed considerable light on the practicality of the CCNW approach for leadership training.

DRUG ABUSE AND THE ABC MODEL

Although certain drug effects of plant-derived substances, such as marijuana, were known by the Chinese as early as 2700 B.C. and opium by the Egyptians by 1500 B.C., the so-called DA (drug abuse) problem, as it presently exists, is historically a twentieth-century phenomenon. Whereas morphinism was recognized as "soldiers illness" following the hypodermic introduction of the narcotic to the wounded during the Civil War, the nature of opiate addiction apparently remained unrecognized by the medical profession as late as 1890, opiate usage at that time being equated with alcohol consumption. It was not until World War

I that the Harrison Act was enacted, thereby making it illegal to purchase narcotics of any kind without a physician's prescription.

In the middle and late 1950's, and certainly during and after the Vietnam War, the emergence of the DA problem became a major social and political issue. At present, the seriousness of the drug problem is attested to by the activity surrounding hospital emergency rooms and police booking agencies. There, it is estimated that from 30 to 50 percent of the injury and homicide victims are drug-related. Various levels of overdosage on a wide range of drugs make up another 10 percent of the cases processed in these facilities. Pushers, ironically called "mothers" on the street, make hundreds, even thousands of dollars daily peddling a variety of drugs to a never-ending multitude of desperate clientele of every age, sex, and social class. Perhaps most egregious are the peddlers loitering around school playgrounds tempting children as young as eight to "get high" on dope of some kind.

So ingrained within our culture has the estimated 8 to 15 percent of the U.S. population that are chronic drug abusers become, a unique "drugese" language has been developed and adopted by this segment of society. For instance, a jargonish lexicon of labels for a wide range of substances found on the street includes: uppers, downers, harry or horse (heroin), footballs (from the shape of diphetamine pills), cartwheels (from the wheel-like scoring on amphetamine tablets), miss emma (morphine), big D (LSD), bluebirds, blue velvet—the list is endless. Also, there is drugese terminology for methods for introduction of various substances: mainlining (intravenous injection), skin popping (epidermal insertion), snorting or blowing snow (inhaling, usually cocaine), and booting (slow intravenous introduction of heroin, allowing it to mix with blood in the eyedropper or syringe), to name a few popular techniques. The problem of diagnosing and treating the drug abuser is even more complicated by the fact that many of these users are "panaddicted," or more appropriately, pandependent, referring to the fact that many different substances and methods of introduction are habitually being used.

Up to this point, the discussion has been about illegal or the so-called street drugs involving the exchange of an estimated $50 billion annually, not to mention the cost in life and limb of drug-related crime and violence. Although perhaps a minor component of the overall drug scene, the overprescription of controlled substances, such as sedatives, antidepressants, and stimulants, as well as the popular minor and major tranquilizers, by well-meaning but overzealous physicians and unscrupulous pharmacists is nonetheless of significance for understanding the drug issue in its totality.

In sum, the enigma of promiscuous drug use has reached such proportions in the U.S. and elsewhere that many politicians, educators, and members of the medical profession have described the drug problem as the number-one social issue of the twentieth century, with the possible exception of the AIDS epidemic of the last decade. The seriousness of the DA situation has not only been recognized in the civilian population, but was also acknowledged by the military in the late 1960's and early 1970's. On the battlefield, as a crewmember of a surface ship, called a "skimmer" by submariners, in the air, or in a deeply submerged submarine, each military person is responsible for the well-being and survival of every other person in the unit. Therefore, any illness or condition, including drug intoxication, that compromises the military person's fitness for duty cannot be tolerated under any circumstances.

Neither incidence nor prevalence statistics for DA is ordinarily widely publicized by the military. However, the incidence of the habitual use of marijuana by the military serving in Vietnam was cited at that time as between 16 and 30 percent. Similar statistics for the submarine service were never made public; however, the fact that a series of five Z-grams (instructions issued by Admiral Zumwalt, Chief of Naval Operations) dealing with various aspects of drug usage by naval personnel was dispersed in rapid order in the 1960's clearly indicated that the problem had been clearly recognized by the U.S. Navy[123].

In response to these Z-grams, two studies of DA in the submarine service were initiated in the early and middle 1970's. The first study compared selected background characteristics of seventy DA cases from the "sub" fleet with a matched control sample of submariners with no history of DA[147]. In general, as compared to the control group, the DA group on average was younger, contained disproportionately more high school dropouts, earned lower scores on the U.S.N. Arithmetical Aptitude Test, and obtained poorer performance grades in submarine school. In addition, their personality test scores showed them to be less emotionally stable, to be more prone to depressive trends, and to be less motivated for submarine duty.

Following up these leads regarding differences in the personality trait patterns of drug abusers in the "sub" service, a second study focused on the personality trait profiles of an independent sample of submariners with a history of DA[153]. The trait profiles were obtained by means of the MMPI, a standardized diagnostic test used extensively by psychiatrists and psychologists in the U.S.

The MMPI contains 435 objective test items, such as "Life is a strain for me most of the time," or "I brood a great deal." The true/false response format is used. There are thirteen subtests, three validity scales, and ten diagnostic scales. A brief descriptive statement regarding each of the subtests follows:

L, or Lie scale, one of three validity scales, measures inordinate deceptive tendencies in responding to the test items; F-scale, tendency to exaggerate symptoms, to malinger; K-scale, tendency to deny symptoms; Hypochondriasis (Hs), over-concern about one's own health; Depression (D), tendency toward depressed mood; Hysteria (Hy), unconscious use of somatic symptoms as anxiety defense mechanisms; Psychopathic Deviate (Pd), tendency toward asocial or dyssocial conduct; Masculinity-feminity (Mf), degree of sex role identification; Paranoia (Pa), excessive suspiciousness, delusional tendencies; Psychasthenia (Pt), characterological or trait anxiety; Schizophrenia (Sc), degree of reality contact; Hypomania (Ma), level of psychic energy; and Social Introversion (Si), tendency for social withdrawal[153].

All MMPI subtest raw scores are customarily transformed to T-scores with a mean of fifty and an SD of ten. The MMPI data in the second submariner study were obtained from four independent groups of males of similar age and background: the navy DA sample, a matched control sample of nonabuser navy men, a sample of nonhospitalized civilian DA's, and finally, a sample of civilian DA's hospitalized in a nearby psychiatric hospital. The MMPI mean subtest profiles are presented in Figure 10.1.

A quote from the summary page of reference[153] succinctly points out the most important conclusions from the profile comparisons. "Overall, the MMPI profiles of the navy drug abuse cases were similar to those of both civilian drug groups, the most prevalent traits being sociopathic in nature. For the navy DA group, the traits of immaturity and social alienation are characteristic, but with little evidence of acute emotional instability. The data indicate that many, if not most, members of the navy drug abuse group may be quite resistive to rehabilitative effort"[153, p. ii].

One further finding, in effect, a working hypothesis, was suggested by certain patterning of the MMPI subtest scores in Figure 10.1. Accordingly, the MMPI patterns for the DA groups suggest two independent "types" of dependencies that, hypothetically at least, might be used to triage DA cases into two groups: those that would be most and those that would be least likely to respond favorably to some sort of therapeutic intervention. The first type is defined by high scores (T-score greater than seventy on "D" (depression subtest), and on "Pt" (psychasthenia), and low scores (T-score less than thirty) on "Ma" (hypomania). This pattern, which appeared to fit the civilian DA groups most closely, was tentatively labeled by the psychoanalytical term "ego-alien." Persons with the ego-alien MMPI pattern are likely to respond favorably to treatment, because their self-perceived DA behavior causes them elevated POSR, especially with an intense −AC component. Simply stated, members of this group feel bad and experience some semblance of guilt about their DA activities. On the other hand, the second MMPI pattern, characterizing the navy DA group in this study, had high peaks on "Pd" (psychopathic deviate), "Sc" (schizophrenia), and "Ma" (hypomania). In addition, the average F-scale score was seventy for this group. Taken together, this pattern suggests the psychoanalytical "ego-syntonic" type, implying that persons with this trait pattern tend to incorporate these traits into their basic personality structure without evoking any significant POSR or −AC. In short, the DA person with this trait pattern appears to like, or at least is complacent, about his or her DA behavior. As a result, the members of this group are less likely to respond beneficially to most kinds of treatment for their drug dependency.

Whereas these two MMPI patterns have only anecdotal evidence for their validity as a triaging strategy, there are some data, perhaps only obliquely related to the DA issue, that the ego-alien and ego-syntonic types as defined by the MMPI do in fact respond differently to chemotherapy for cancerous tumors[44]. That is, the life expectancy for cancer patients with ego-syntonic MMPI pattern

Figure 10.1
MMPI Profiles for the Submariner DA and Control Group and Two Civilian DA Groups

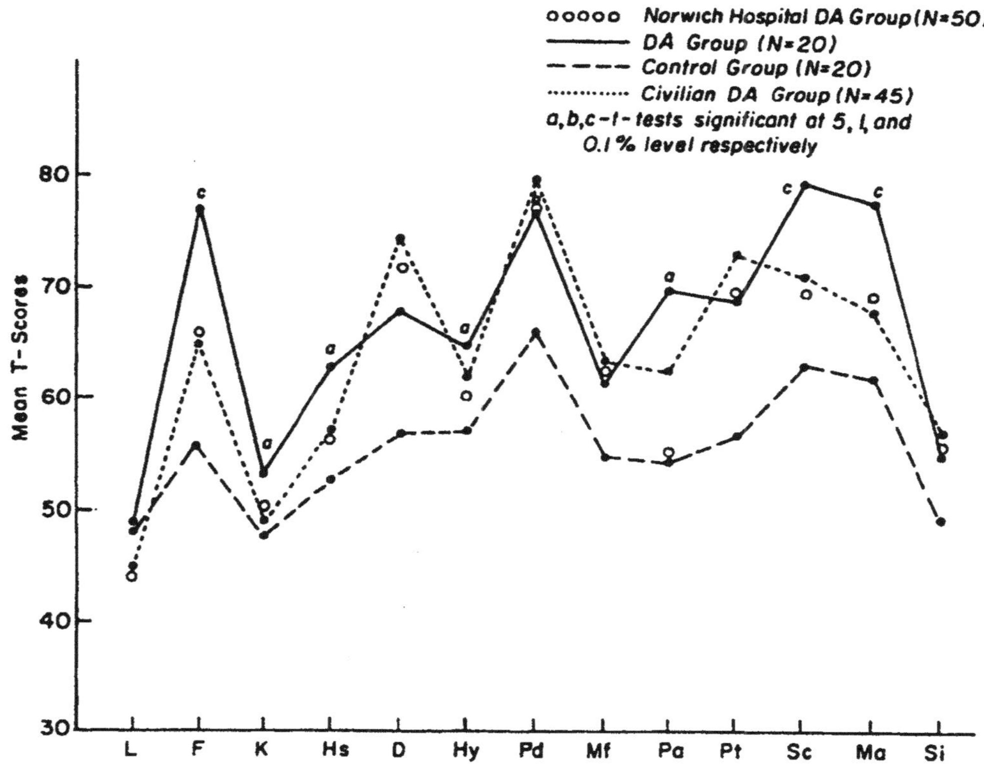

treated with cancer-fighting chemicals may be three to five times longer than for persons with the same type of cancer undergoing the same chemotherapeutic treatment but with the ego-alien MMPI pattern [153]. Note, this finding is the reverse of the treatment triaging dichotomy, that is, persons with the ego-alien personalities are likely to be better therapeutic prospects for treatment than are drug-dependent persons with the ego-syntonic personalities. Although admittedly a speculative hypothesis but possibly of heuristic value, there may be a meaningful relationship among stress reactivity (POSR), proneness for drug dependency, and the efficiency of the immune system in fighting cancer.

In order to follow up this speculative hypothesis and fully aware that observations based on a sample of one are only suggestive, a true anecdote may be helpful. The author was closely associated with a Captain (M.D.) in the submarine service whose MMPI profile corresponded closely with the ego-syntonic pattern. After retiring from the service, this physician developed an inoperable oat-cell tumor, generally described by cancer specialists as having a 99 percent probability of being terminal within two years. This submarine physician lived a relatively healthy life before his death, thirteen years after the cancer diagnosis.

Before introducing some possible "ABC solutions" to certain aspects of the DA problem and before looking at some of the treatment approaches that have been and are still being used, clarification of two terms found throughout the DA literature would seem to be in order. One such term is "addiction." The former surgeon general, Dr. C. Everett Koop, has repeatedly insisted that habitual smoking of cigarettes is the result of an *addiction* to the drug nicotine found in tobacco. However, this use of the word addiction is inconsistent with the recommendation of the WHO's (World Health Organization's) thirteenth report on addiction-producing drugs in 1964. The unequivocal recommendation in this report was that the expression addiction be dropped because it is "too general and imprecise." It recommends instead that the expression "drug dependence" be substituted in all cases for the word addiction used in this context.

Following this proclamation by WHO, the important fact was raised by experts in the DA field that different drugs generally cause two distinct types of dependencies: physical dependence or psychological dependence. Physical dependency results from the pharmacodynamic action of certain drugs taken in high dosages for long periods of time. As a result, biochemical and neurophysiological changes occur such that a stereotyped set of withdrawal symptoms unique to the particular drug occurs when its use is stopped. For example, the withdrawal syndrome resulting from opiate or barbiturate dependence consists of such symptoms as anxiety, restlessness, yawning, fever, dehydration, cramps, nausea, and excessive weight loss. Although supportive psychological treatment is recommended as an adjunct, treatment of the physically dependent person is essentially a medical matter and, therefore, is beyond the scope of this book.

On the other hand, psychological dependency, wholly within the purview of this book, is defined as a persistent craving for the euphoria, stimulation, tranquilization, hallucinations, and other pleasurable mental effects (+AC) or, as an Italian might say, *la dolce vita* produced by the ingestion or injection of certain drugs. Withdrawal from substances producing psychological dependence, especially CNS stimulants, although not producing any remarkable physical symptoms, may result in deep, intrinsic depression. Examples of drugs tending to produce psychological dependence are: cocaine and its derivative "crack," marijuana, hashish, amphetamines, and LSD.

Therapy for persons who are psychologically dependent on an array of drugs is carried out by both physicians as well as by nonmedical professionals, such as specialized clinical psychologists. The specific therapeutic techniques used vary from patient to patient, and depend upon the length of the dependency, the general health status of the patient, and the type of drug involved.

Generally speaking, conventional approaches for the treatment of psychological drug dependency consist of one or more IVP's presented in Table 8.2. These IVP's can be grouped into three broad categories: ego-supportive (IVP's numbered 2, 3, 8, and 9 in Table 8.2), behavioral modification (IVP's 10 through 16), and attitude change (IVP's 1, 2, 6, 8, and 10).

Sometimes overlooked in the application of some of these therapeutic approaches is the critical point of the drug dependency issue, namely, that the questions of the etiology, perseveration, and elimination of the drug-dependent behavior must be focused upon in its entirety. The fundamental assumption underlying the discussion of these three aspects of the dependency issue is that the root cause of DA is stress, or, more appropriately, POSR. Enter the ABC model of stress.

In the first place, the expression "drug problem," which was viewed by the federal government as so critical that a cabinet level (so-called) drug czar was appointed, is a misnomer. It is not a *drug problem*; it is a *people* problem. The National Rifle Association argues that guns do not kill or maim anyone; rather, it is irresponsible, sometimes irrational, *people* misusing guns who cause the injuries and homicides in such huge numbers. Similarly, securely packaged "crack" cocaine, so popular on the street, or opiates in any form are harmless. The focus should therefore be upon the dynamics of the *people* who compulsively ingest or inject these dangerous substances.

Looking at the ABC model of stress in Figure 3.1 it becomes necessary to raise several questions regarding the DA issue, questions for which answers, or a least some degree of enlightenment, are to be sought from the implications of the model. First, in Phase I of the model, what NPP's underlie the drive (energy mobilization in Phase II) that leads to the selection in Phase III of the dependency-producing contingencies, which, in turn, bring about a drug-dependent state? To begin with, a partial answer to the question has to do with the fact that the NPP's involved in drug dependency generally consist of secondary, mainly social, needs (affiliation, affection, and status, for instance), since few, if any, drugs satisfy primary needs, such as need for food, fluid, or breathing air. Since social needs develop mainly by learning processes in the early developmental stages, the burden of providing opportunities for the establishment of socially acceptable NPP's falls upon educational activities carried out in homes and institutions. The goals of these educational endeavors should be to establish a socially adaptable value hierarchy associated with these needs together with an array of PRC's and ARC's for satisfying each need. For example, the value of the NAch should be emphasized in educational institutions and home settings[78]. The reinforcement contingencies for satisfaction of NAch could then be spelled out along career and vocational lines.

Second, in Phase III, the environmental antecedents or activators become the means by which mobilized energy or drive, underpinned by prevailing NPP's, take on the directional properties of motivational vectors. What are some of these activators that lead to the selection and development of drug-dependent contingencies supported by these NPP's? To start with, the influence of peers and pushers is an important component of the "A" phase in the ABC model. Although less overt perhaps, there are also such factors as the boredom and persistent negative affect (−AC) often resulting from the potential drug user's perceptions of his or her own sometimes hopeless life situation. A preadolescent or adolescent, homeless for years, wandering around searching for a set of contingencies (PRC's and ARC's) that will reduce the unrelenting −AC is an example of the environmental circumstances in which peers and pushers function very compellingly as activators. In other words, POSR, caused by the absence of effective PRC's and ARC's for strong needs, may themselves become activators for the development and maintenance of drug-dependent behavior. Once begun, these contingencies are sustained by RF− (the avoidance of −AC by the contingency of using drugs). In addition, the so-called "chaining" and "shaping" mechanisms associated with the "A" phase come into play. For example, pressure from peers and pushers in the context of an environmental event (a rock concert, for instance) may result in enhancement of the intensity of the motivation to try drugs.

In the third place, the "B" or feedforward sequence of the ABC model becomes the dependency-producing contingency for satisfying the prevailing NPP(s). These motivational vectors can be both positive and negative, approach or avoidance, at least during the early stages of the development of a drug-dependent condition. The positively valent motives can be carried out by contingencies selected as a means to satisfy the social needs described above; however, after experiencing the euphoria, the so-called "high," and the renewed self-confidence that some drugs produce, the goal of repeating this experience takes on increased positive valence. Moreover, the negatively valent or avoidance motives with their associated drug-consuming contingencies serve to reduce at least temporarily the POSR, in particular, the −AC component. Thus, RF− becomes an important factor in this compulsive behavior. Taken together, these positive and negative motives, satisfied by drug-use contingencies, are supported by a variety of RF+ and RF− reinforcers, and, all too often, by insufficient Pu+ and Pu− outcomes or "C" events. As a result, the OR, the expectancy of $RF^{\pm}/Pu^{\pm}$, is greatly increased by drug-taking contingencies. For example, one of the author's patients, hopelessly dependent on high dosages of marijuana for many years, came up with the following proposition: "show me a quick-acting way that I can gain the complete confidence in myself, the delightful 'high' I get and the almost instantaneous disassociation from all of my problems that I get from smoking four or five joints, and I will stop smoking pot forever." Therein is the persistent dilemma that every therapist in the DA field continually faces.

Fourth, the "C" or outcome sequence for the ABC model is one of the major forces controlling the development, modification, or elimination of the learning processes resulting in the perseverance of the dependency-producing PRC's and ARC's. For the drug-dependent person, these PRC's and ARC's become the one and only set of contingencies by which the dominating NPP's can be satisfied. Stated differently, these learned drug-dependency contingencies become compulsive behaviors by which the OR will be sustained or enhanced.

Fifth, another compelling force affecting both the development and persistence of drug-dependent behavior is the effect of feedbackward processes, both intrinsic and extrinsic. As discussed earlier in the section on creativity and POSR, intrinsic or internal feedback, both positive and negative, is experiential and results from the person's self-perception of the consequences of the completion of a series of contingencies. Examples of positive and negative intrinsic feedback for the drug-dependent person are the drug-induced euphoric high and the withdrawal depression in the same order. It may be further recalled that extrinsic feedback, both positive and negative, is external and results from the backaction of the environment, usually social in nature, to the drug-dependent behavior. Positive extrinsic feedback for drug-dependent activity usually comes from pushers and other drug-dependent persons. Negative extrinsic feedback, on the other hand, generally has its origin from the segment of society, including government, that opposes DA in any form. Consistent with the "Law of Effect," positive feedback, both extrinsic and intrinsic, results in the entrenchment of a given set of drug-dependent contingencies, whereas negative feedback, extrinsic and intrinsic, only to a certain extent, tends to modify or eliminate drug-dependent behavior (*see* the discussion of Pu− in Chapter 3).

It is seen in the ABC model that feedbackward processes may from time to time effect changes in the predominant NPP(s). These changes in the NPP(s) would of course transfer to changes in drive level and eventually to changes in the contingencies selected to satisfy the prevailing NPP. For example, the author was familiar with the case history of a young man, a high school valedictorian, who, upon graduation, was unable to find satisfactory employment. During the same period, he was asked by his parents to find his own living accommodations, to put it euphemistically. Because of the high-IED produced by the accumulative effect of these high-SEP stressors, rejection and unemployment, this young man became hopelessly "hooked" on a strong CNS stimulant, methamphetamine, called AMT on the street. For a time, the drug-use contingency and associated behavior served to reduce the intensity of the POSR caused by the high-IED situation. The pleasurable euphoric high in addition to the POSR reduction, in particular the −AC element, resulting from taking the AMT quickly resulted in an overpowering psychological dependency requiring increasingly higher dosages to obtain the same effect. Finally, paranoid delusions, chronic insomnia, and combativeness necessitated his hospitalization. Deep depression, unresponsive to antidepressant medication, occurred during withdrawal. During psychotherapy, the patient, reminded of his academic prowess in high school, was assisted by the therapist in obtaining a substantial scholarship to a nearby university. Sometime later, it became evident that the compelling NPP had changed from the need to reduce the intensity of POSR and experience the pleasant "high" produced by AMT to an NPP dominated by NAch[80]. Contingencies appropriate for entering and pursuing a degree program in the university were adopted and the drug use stopped. Thus, the negative feedback from a "bad trip" plus supportive therapy had produced a new, much more adaptive, NPP.

Based upon the implications of the ABC model expressed above, some suggestions for the prevention and, if need be, treatment of drug dependency follow: (1) mainly by educational means, attempt in the early developmental stages to ensure that socially acceptable needs (NAch or affiliation, for example) are represented in the prevalent NPP's, particularly for dependency-prone individuals (those from broken homes and substandard socioeconomic settings, for instance); (2) once the drive level, supported by these NPP's, takes on directional characteristics, introduce and reinforce socially adaptable contingencies for these NPP's; (3) identify the high-SEP stressors by means of SIRO in order to surmount those barriers likely to impede or block these contingencies. As a consequence, the IED will be diminished together with a correlated reduction in the associated POSR; (4) implement appropriate IVP's for these high-SEP stressors; (5) provide ample positive feedback and minimal negative feedback so that the desirable NPP's will be fully nurtured, and, in the long run, sustained. As a result of these endeavors, an adaptable value system will emerge, and effective drug-free PRC's and ARC's will develop, thus significantly enhancing the OR's associated with these reinforcement contingencies; and, finally, (6) having maintained the POSR within acceptable limits of intensity by identifying, and then overcoming, the major high-SEP stressors, be vigilant in protecting the developing person from activators (the "A" in ABC) (peers and pushers, for example). In this way, it will be possible to avoid the implementation of dependency-producing contingencies as a means of adjusting to the inevitable occasions when accumulative POSR approach debilitative intensity levels.

CAUSES OF WARS AND THE ABC MODEL

War, like suicide, is an attempt at an immediate solution to a long-standing problem. In some ways, war in geopolitics is like surgery in medicine: Sometimes trauma must be inflicted upon healthy tissue in order to arrest, control, or cure an injury or a disease process. As the title of this chapter implies, the causes of wars, the *casus belli*, are to be found from an examination of a sequence of interrelated events occurring over varying time intervals preceding the actual onset of hostilities. In short, the causes of war are initiated, develop, and unfold during peacetime.

For example, decades before the "shot heard around the world" at Lexington to start the Revolutionary War, the colonists in the Boston area were expressing their resentment of British rule with great vigor. The Boston Tea Party, "no taxation without representation," and "give me liberty or give me death" all attest to the intensity of the emotional reactivity of the patriots in those times. In the language of the ABC model, were SIRO data have been available from a sample of those colonists, a preponderance of stressors related to high taxes, suppression of their freedom and the like would have undoubtedly received very high SEP ratings. In other words, the IED and associated POSR would have been very intense for many of the patriots at that time.

It would seem to be a valid assumption that similar sequences of these predispositional factors had occurred prior to each of the eight or so major wars in which the U.S. participated since the Declaration of Independence was signed in 1776. One thinks, for instance, of the predispositional factors related to the slavery issue leading to the Civil War, of the questions regarding colonization resulting in the Spanish-American War, of America's support of Chiang Kai-shek's democratic movement against the Chinese communists, and, after that, against the Japanese, culminating in Pearl Harbor and World War II. Similarly, the Iran-Contra affair and the munitions sales of the U.S., Germany, France, and Russia to Iraq are considered to have contributed to Saddam Hussein's invasion of Kuwait, to be followed five months later by Operation Desert Storm.

Since predispositional factors for wars generally develop slowly over considerable lengths of time, they are more accessible to preventive strategies than are precipitating factors for wars, that is, circumscribed events that suddenly, and often unexpectedly, exacerbate hostilities. Examples of precipitating factors for wars are readily apparent in almost all wars: the assassination of the Archduke Ferdinand and his wife to start World War I, Pearl Harbor to trigger the U.S. entry into World War II, and recently, Iraq's invasion of Kuwait to touch off Operation Desert Shield progressing to Operation Desert Storm. As stated above, however, precipitating factors are symptoms or by-products of the unfolding of many predispositional factors, and, as such, are less amenable to the preventive principles suggested by the ABC model.

In sum, in the language of the ABC model, the causes of wars are many and varied. In general, the hypothesis being entertained is that the predominant cause of war is the build up of POSR in the decision-making bodies as well as the citizenry of one geopolitical organization caused by the blockage of their goal-directed activities by the barriers (stressors) imposed by another geopolitical group (see Figure 3.1). It should be recalled that the channeled energy represented by the motivational vectors in Figures 2.1 and 3.1 is underpinned by a number of prepotent needs, the need profiles (NPP's), of each group. Should the reinforcement contingencies for the NPP's of potential combatant A, for example, be blocked or impeded by the barriers (stressors) imposed by combatant B (or vice versa), then possible PRC's and ARC's for these needs become obscure or nonexistent (*see* Equation 4.3). In lay language, neither side has a way out. A no-win situation for both parties has been created[84].

As a result of this latent or sometimes manifest intergroup conflict, avoidance motivation and associated negative, intergroup attitudes proliferate on both sides[50]. Although avoidance contingencies may temporarily control the POSR intensity level, until the barriers are removed or are made more permeable, the IED generated for both potential combatants will remain high. Lack of communication and absence of attempts at conflict resolution tend to sustain the so-called cold war atmosphere.

The above description of selected aspects of the ABC model that apply to the dynamics of warfare suggests several general principles for preventing predispositional factors from progressing to precipitating events with war an inevitable eventuality in many cases.

Principles for the Prevention of Wars

The following principles are derived from the ABC model (Figures 2.1 and 3.1) as expanded in Equations 4.1, 4.2, and 4.3.

WPP-1 (War Preventive Principle 1). Figure 2.1 and Table 5.1 suggest that conflicts, defined as motivational vectors in opposition, may in fact be a special class of high-SEP stressors. Therefore, persons in the governmental positions of the interacting nations should be vigilant in detecting the onset of these conflicts, generally signaled by intense POSR within a significant segment of the decision makers of the nations concerned.

WPP-2 (War Preventive Principle 2). Having identified the signs and symptoms of international conflict, preferably in its latent stage, examine the cultures of the two or more groups involved to identify the most prepotent needs underpinning the intersecting motivational vectors causing the conflict. Then, with the major prepotent needs on both sides of the conflict identified, consider the dynamics of these needs. That is, focus on the nature of the reinforcement contingencies associated with these needs. For example, the need for power of competing nations often supports continuous intense striving for material or territorial gain by means of exploitation of adjacent countries[63, 79].

WPP-3 (War Preventive Principle 3). With the major prepotent needs and the correlated reinforcement contingencies of the conflicting nations identified, collect SIRO data from a sample of high-ranking decision makers on both sides of the conflict. These SIRO data should delineate the stressors (barriers) with the highest SEP, stressors that are blocking the PRC's and ARC's for the prepotent needs of one or both of the potential combatants.

WPP-4 (War Preventive Principle 4). Determine the sources and nature of these stressors (blockages) as well as their degree of permeability. Identify and prioritize the most appropriate reinforcement contingencies for surmounting them.

WPP-5 (War Preventive Principle 5). Select and implement the most effective IVP's (Table 8.2) aimed at reducing the SEP of these localized stressors as well as those IVP's focused upon decreasing the level of the IED at the interface between the potential belligerents. In general, IVP's numbered 22, 23, 24, 26, 29, and 30 in Table 8.2 or some modifications of some one or another of them are recommended for this purpose.

By coincidence, this chapter was written during Operation Desert Shield/Desert Storm in the fall and winter of 1990–91. It would seem timely (as the chapter title suggests) to look backward to ascertain to what degree the application of the ABC-based preventive principles described above might have prevented this destructive war.

WPP-1 enjoins world watchers everywhere to be surveillant in identifying the origin of conflict stressors and the correlated POSR among the decision makers of militant geopolitical organizations. For example, in Iraq, Saddam Hussein assumed the presidency in 1979. Similar to other megalomaniacal dictators, such as Nicolae Ceausescu of Romania and the Shah of Iran, he immediately launched a brutal purge of his inner circle of military officers and Baath Party officials. Dozens of officers, even five of the twenty-two members of the governing Revolutionary Command Council, were summarily executed. The U.S. government and the United Nations in concert vehemently registered their objections to this inhumane behavior. POSR were unquestionably very intense on all sides.

Having identified this intense international conflict, WPP-2 recommends that an examination of the cultures of the two (or more) conflicting groups be carried out in order to delineate the prepotent need(s) underpinning the motivational vectors accounting for the conflict.

Dictatorships, in terms of the cultural context from which they arise, are the most simple form of government in the sense that the executive, legislative, and judicial functions of a multicameral, pluralistic democracy are all subsumed by one person, in the case of Iraq, by Saddam Hussein. Therefore, an assessment of the personality of Hussein should describe the NPP of the government of that country. Personality specialists who have studied this dictator use such trait descriptors as paranoid, megalomanic, messianic, psychopathic, egocentric, vicious, sadistic, and aggressive to describe his prevailing trait configuration. One psychologist who studied Saddam in depth diagnosed him as suffering from "malignant narcissism, defined as a personality disorder with associated traits of grandiosity, paranoia, and ruthlessness."

David McClelland, one of the foremost authorities on the subject of human motivation, has developed and partially validated a theory containing the proposition that there are three major needs basic for human motivation: affiliation, achievement, and power[78, 79]. Power is defined in this context as the capacity to influence and control the people, and, to an extent, people-related events in the immediate environment[79]. The greater the control, the greater the power.

Once attained, Hussein's power has been and still is being maintained by fear, coercion, and intimidation.

In ABC terms, what were the sources of Saddam's power that produced the mobilized energy for such intense, sharply focused motivational vectors? One major source of power was his unchallenged capacity to impose reward and punishment for complete submission and for nonallegiance, respectively. Another source of power, especially effective in the Islamic world, was his ability to convincingly project a messianic or liberator image to his people. Based upon the documented history of the homicidal purge at the outset of his presidency, upon his bloody attack on Iran in September 1980, upon his lethal use of toxic gas on his own population, and, finally, upon his unprovoked occupation of Kuwait on August 2, 1990, it would seem obvious that the initiation and implementation of this brutal behavior resulted from the prepotency of the need for power and self-aggrandizement.

In addition to the identification of the prepotent needs of the conflicting groups as a requirement of WPP-2, it is also necessary to evaluate the reinforcement contingencies by means of which these needs are characteristically being satisfied. In the case of Saddam Hussein, obviously the need for power and control of the masses was intense; therefore, it would be expected that the reinforcement contingencies for that compelling need would be supported by tremendous amounts of channeled energy. Moreover, in the Moslem society in particular, despots, including monarchs, typically maintain their positions (that is, satisfy their need for power) not only by subjugating their own people, but also by repeatedly demonstrating their unchallenged role as a protector of the people and as a conqueror of any nation that appears to challenge their authority. Accordingly, in 1980, Saddam attacked Iran, and, after eight bloody but futile years ended the war by producing the grand finale of blasting Teheran with his newly acquired SCUD missiles. Thus, by terminating the war that he was not winning with this "big bang," so to speak, in 1988, he saw himself as increasing the image of his being a savior from the infidel, Iran, and from Zionism—a true conqueror. Thus, his need for power was at least temporarily reinforced.

Two years passed, after which Saddam's drive (mobilized energy) underpinned by his intense need for power and prestige again increased and became more focused. With a modern army of a million men, 700 high-performance aircraft, 3,000 battle tanks and troop carriers plus thousands of SCUD missiles, he must have reasoned that it was time to demonstrate his prowess once more. So, recalling Egypt's crushing defeat by the highly efficient Israeli military in 1967, Saddam again must have reasoned that the oil-rich, tiny nation of Kuwait (with a population of less than 3 million) was a natural attack point.

One requirement of WPP-2 was not, but should have been, acted upon during the interim between the end of the Iran/Iraq war in 1988 and the occupation of Kuwait on August 2, 1990. That is, the prevailing activity during the eight years of the Iran/Iraq war demonstrated clearly that the major reinforcement contingencies for Saddam's intense need for power centered around intimidation, exploitation, and destruction of weaker nations proximal to Iraq. Thus, the one requirement of WPP-2 that should have been implemented during this eight-year time frame was that once the reinforcement contingencies for Saddam's power need had been identified and assessed, this information should have been used as a criterion for early detection of any war-provoking activity during the 1988–90 war-free period. Incidentally, it is interesting to note that the tiny, new nation of Israel had noted and reported Iraq's intense mobilization for conquest during this same time span—but to no avail.

In sum, had the provisions of WPP-2 been considered, certain members of the U.N. Security Council, the U.S. Congress, and other world leaders should have been able to predict some sort of aggressive, brutal, and self-serving behavior from Saddam Hussein, even though the specific intrusion and occupation of Kuwait would not necessarily have been identified as his prime target.

WPP-3 recommends the collection of SIRO data from a sample of decision-makers on both sides of the international conflict, the purpose of this procedure being to localize possible barriers or stressors imposed by each potential adversary upon the other's goal-directed activity. SIRO data collected at that time from Tariq Aziz, prime minister of Iraq, for example, would quite likely show such stressors as "OPEC's cap on oil prices," "Israel's expansionism," and "the arrogance of the Kuwaiti royalty" as having very high SEP's. On the other hand, a SIRO provided by Yitzhak Shamir, then prime minister of Israel, would probably yield such high-SEP stressors as "PLO terrorism," "Iraq's nuclear potential," and "housing for the Russian immigrants." WPP-4 is an extension of WPP-3 in that it recommends that for each of the stressors delineated by the application of SIRO as required by WPP-3, it is necessary to determine which of the potential combatants is responsible for initiating and sustaining the elevated SEP of each specific stressor.

The problem was that in the late 1970's, the U.S. and Iran (not Iraq) were engaged in a deep-seated conflict over the 22 American hostages incarcerated for more than 400 days by the Ayatollah Khomeini. In this situation, F. Heider's Balance Theory of intergroup attitudes came into play[50]. This theory simply states that positive and negative interpersonal and intergroup attitudes tend to change polarity until an equilibrated tension state within the group is reached. Accordingly, the U.S. tended to have positive attitudes toward Iraq because, at that time, Iraq, being at war with Iran, held intense negative attitudes toward that country, the same nation toward which the U.S. held similarly intense negative attitudes because of the hostage situation. This interrelationship might be expressed very well by the time-worn aphorism, "My enemy's enemy is my very good friend." Thus, as recommended by WPP-3, the SIRO data collected from the U.S. Department of Defense in the 1979–81 period would likely have shown the highest SEP stressors to be associated with the Iran hostage situation and not with any conflict relationship with Iraq. In effect then, the high IED stemming from the Iran hostage problem had masked the potential stressors related to the Iraqi situation.

WPP-5 suggests that, with the prepotent needs and the correlated reinforcement contingencies of the conflicting groups delineated, and, with the major intergroup stressors localized, appropriate IVP's should be selected and applied. There is one overriding principle that should be brought to bear when attempting to solve intergroup conflict, namely, "avoid, if at all possible, allowing the conflict resolution process to become a zero-sums game, that is, a we win/you lose (or vice versa) outcome." Thus, the two most appropriate IVP's for resolving conflicts at the international level are likely to be Kurt Lewin's FFA (Force Field Analysis) and the ICRP (Intergroup Conflict Resolution Procedure), both listed in Table 8.2, as IVP's 36 and 29, respectively.

The first step in resolving an intergroup conflict, most certainly at an international level, is to conduct an FFA to ascertain which of two possible biases exists in the relationship between the opposing motivational vectors of the groups involved[70, 116]. Stated differently, the purpose of FFA is to determine whether the opposing forces are at equilibrium, or are approaching it, or whether there is a significant imbalance of the opposing forces in one direction or another. In the first instance, wherein the opposing forces are balanced, an ICRP should be applied for the purpose of reducing the intensity level of the POSR within or between the conflicting groups. In group conflict situations in which the potential outcome is so serious as to result in warfare, the primary goal of an ICRP is to arrive at some sort of a compromise solution, so that both potential combatants receive some semblance of positive reinforcement for their blocked goal-directed activity. A timely example of this proposed conflict solution might be the division of some disputed land area, such as the strategically and economically important Kurile Islands, presently occupied by Russia but hotly contested by Japan. Consistent with the ABC model, this approach to conflict resolution should result in a significant reduction in the intensity of POSR on both sides, since the intergroup barriers or stressors would have been partially removed. As a result, the IED between the intersecting groups should be greatly reduced, thus making the occurrence of a full-blown confrontation less likely.

An example of a fairly balanced or impasse conflict situation functioning at a high-IED level would be the relationship between Iraq and Israel in the early 1980's. It may be recalled that Israel apparently anticipated that if Saddam Hussein were to develop a deliverable nuclear bomb, being a megalomaniacal tyrant, he would try to shift the equilibrium of forces in the region in his direction by "nuking" Israel back into the stone age. Therefore, to avoid this eventuality, Israel "took out" Saddam's nuclear facilities in 1981, the result being a re-establishment of the pre-existing balanced conflict condition, but this time at a much lower IED level. Interestingly, the Israeli press in reporting the event at that time characterized the raid on Baghdad as a neutralization mission, consistent with the theoretical basis for the FFA procedure.

Perhaps a more proximal example of an equilibrated yet high-IED conflict situation between two of the most militarily powerful nations on earth was the cold war relationship between the Soviet Union and the United States since World War II. The IVP that apparently sustained relative peace during this time frame was the arms race wherein the armamentarium of each country acted as a strong deterrent against the outbreak of warfare initiated by the other side.

In the second case in which the resultant of the two motivational vectors had shifted strongly in one direction or another, the IVP for this imbalanced conflict situation should be directed toward either reducing the motivational vectors on the strong side of the conflict or by increasing the intensity of the vectors on the weak side–or a combination of both strategies. Combined or singly, this approach to conflict resolution should significantly reduce the POSR of the participants involved, as well as lower the IED intensity at the conflict interface.

One example of this approach to equalizing an imbalanced conflict situation is the arming by the U.S. of the Afghan rebels opposing the Russian-supported Kabul government of Afghanistan. A second example of this imbalanced conflict condition may be found in the relationship between Iraq and Iran in the 1980's–Iraq with a highly trained, "high-tech" military and Iran with a "ragtag" horde of untrained adolescents, truly a David and Goliath situation. Mentioned earlier was the fact that even though duly warned by Israel that Saddam was likely to lash out at some weaker nation after the Iran war ended, neither the United States nor the United Nations attempted to take measures to prevent the Iraqi arms buildup. In retrospect, as discussed earlier, one of the reasons the U.S. was passive in this matter was that the congruence of Iraq's and the U.S.'s negative attitudes toward Iran during the hostage crisis was still strong. As a result, moderately strong *positive* attitudes toward Iraq were sustained throughout this time frame. Thus, the imbalanced conflict situation between Iraq and Iran was sustained.

The dictates of WPP-5 suggest that the United Nations Security Council should have appointed a committee to investigate and rebuke countries, such as France, Germany, Russia, and the United States, for selling advanced weaponry to Saddam Hussein, thus assisting him in building the third largest military machine in the world. In this manner, Saddam's seemingly insatiable need for power would have lacked adequate PRC's and ARC's for him to even attempt to carry out the egregious campaign against Kuwait. As a result, Desert Shield followed by Desert Storm would not have been necessary.

In sum, wars are caused by a series of predispositional events occurring during peacetime usually followed by some precipitating event or series of events. The high intensity of the POSR among the decision makers of the two or more potential combatant groups is symptomatic of an existing or impending intergroup conflict. Defined as motivational vectors in opposition, this conflict situation causes the level of IED between the intersecting groups to increase significantly. To resolve these conflicts, it is first necessary to identify the prepotent needs and the correlated reinforcement contingencies of the possible adversaries. Second, barriers or more appropriately high-SEP stressors, imposed by either side upon the other must also be identified by SIRO or other means and removed or made more permeable. As a result, the IED between the conflicting groups is thereby reduced. Thereupon the propensity for war is significantly diminished.

11
A Brief Summary

It has been said, "Death and taxes will always be with us, but death, at least, doesn't get any worse." The IED's for most of us, however, seem to worsen steadily because of such high-SEP stressors as international conflict, overpopulation, educational deficiencies, demise of the family unit, illness, crime, drugs, and AIDS. The ABC model of stress was never meant to be a panacea, but, hopefully, the model may cause the big research guns in the field of stress to re-aim their volleys on the most important aspect of the phenomena. Stress is *not* heat, cold, obnoxious bosses, illnesses, or failure. These are environmental *stressors*, impediments or barriers to goal-directed behavior. The SEP of these stressors must be assessed, of course. SIRO does that very well. However, the dynamics of stress, or POSR, caused by these stressors should be the refocused target. Equation 4.1, POSR = K(IED/AR), delineates these dynamics quite well.

In the 1930's, Kurt Lewin sounded the wake-up call by pointing out the directional and time-dimensional aspects of behavior, symbolized by vectors[68]. "ABC" goes further to indicate that certain impediments or barriers (stressors) of different degrees of permeability interfere with these goal-directed vectors, causing the POSR.

Accordingly, from "ABC" emanate three stress-preventive recommendations: (1) identify the high-SEP stressors making up the high-IED situation of concern, preferably by means of SIRO; (2) once these stressors have been identified, develop maximally effective PRC's and ARC's to overcome them; and (3) control the intensity level of POSR by enhancing the AR by educational or other means.

The expected result will be a significant drop in the intensity of the POSR and a substantial enhancement of overall SCC.

Among the academicians in the Ivy League, it is a well-known fact that Professor Albert Einstein had little use, to put it euphemistically, for chemists.

He is said to have said, "The problem with chemists is that chemistry is too hard for them." This might very well be the same problem for the many experts working in the area of stress. The topic of stress might be too hard for us. The ABC model of stress, however, represents at least one feeble attempt to simplify the problem of understanding stress for the layman and the professional alike.

Using our capacity for psychoimagery, an unembellished scenario for the "ABC" frame of reference for the topic of stress might be: YOU RECEIVE AN URGENT REQUEST TO GO TO A NEARBY TOWN *(A)*. THOUGHTFULLY, YOU CHOOSE THE SAFEST AND MOST DIRECT ROUTE TO THE TOWN (RF CONTINGENCY SELECTION). HURRIEDLY, YOU DRIVE DOWN THAT ROAD *(B)*. SUDDENLY, YOU COME UPON A ROADBLOCK (A HIGH-SEP STRESSOR). CLEARLY, THE SIGNS AND SYMPTOMS OF POSR (STRESS) APPEAR. FRUSTRATED (−AC), YOU STUDY THE BARRIER, LOOKING FOR WAYS TO GO AROUND IT, GO THROUGH IT, OR MOVE IT OUT OF YOUR WAY. YOU DO ONE OF THESE. IT WORKS. THE POSR DISSIPATES (SCC). ANTICIPATIVE, YOU CONTINUE DOWN THE ROAD. RELIEVED, YOU ARRIVE AT YOUR DESTINATION *(C)* (RF+, +AC). THIS IS THE ABC MODEL OF STRESS.

Appendix A
PIB (Personal Inventory Barometer)

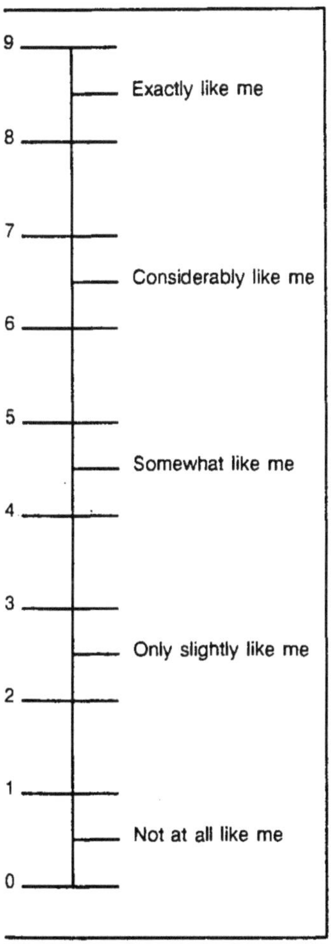

1	2	3	4	5
6	7	8	9	10
11	12	13	14	15
16	17	18	19	20
21	22	23	24	25
26	27	28	29	30
31	32	33	34	35
36	37	38	39	40
41	42	43	44	45
46	47	48	49	50

Appendix B
Affective Response Inventory

Research Code No.#____

INSTRUCTIONS: Please try to recall and develop a mental image of one situation in the past when you were exposed to a set of very high-SEP stressors. Then concentrating on that situation, please check (V) a point on the bi-polar scales below, the check to correspond to how you FELT at that time and in that situation. Try to be as frank and honest as possible. Your responses are CONFIDENTIAL. Further, there is no time limit, so take your time. THANKS VERY MUCH FOR YOUR COOPERATION.

	...1...2...3...4...5...6...7...8...9...	
1. unafraid	... ...	afraid
2. miserable	... ...	contented
3. angry	... ...	delighted
4. glad	... ...	furious
5. vindictive	... ...	non-vindictive
6. vicious	... ...	benevolent
7. strong	... ...	weak
8. dissatisfied	... ...	satisfied
9. calm	... ...	upset
10. trusting	... ...	suspicious
11. constructive	... ...	destructive
12. unconfident	... ...	confident
13. cold	... ...	hot
14. displeased	... ...	pleased
15. rested	... ...	tired
16. friendly	... ...	unfriendly
17. unconfused	... ...	confused
18. relaxed	... ...	tense
19. heart-palpitating	... ...	no palpitating
20. annoyed	... ...	untroubled
21. turned-on	... ...	turned-off
22. trembling	... ...	steady
23. bored stiff	... ...	enthused
24. dry-mouthed	... ...	salivating
25. unanxious	... ...	anxious
26. happy	... ...	sad
27. euphoric	... ...	depressed
28. unprovoked	... ...	provoked
29. blushing	... ...	pale
30. palms sweaty	... ...	palms dry

FINALLY, please check <u>a</u> point on the timeline BELOW corresponding approximately to how long ago the situation you recalled had in fact occurred. <u>THANKS AGAIN</u>.

1 week or less	1 month	1-6 months	6 mo-1 yr	1-2 yrs	2-3 years	more than 3 years

Appendix C
Weybrew Activity Inventory

Research Code No.#____

INSTRUCTIONS: Please check (√) ONE of the blanks of each of the following statements as to how characteristic this behavior is of you day-in-and-day-out.

Always or Almost always	Occasionally	Never	
1.____	____	____	1. On a moving escalator, walk up the steps to get to the top more quickly.
2.____	____	____	2. At a stoplight, while waiting for the red light to change, "inch" your car forward to gain a few feet.
3.____	____	____	3. At the office or work place, generally feel that you won't have enough time to finish your work.
4.____	____	____	4. Almost anywhere or anytime, I'm inclined to keep looking at my watch to check on the time.
5.____	____	____	5. At both workplace and home, prepare daily, a detailed schedule of what must be done, purchases to be made, phone calls to be completed, etc.
6.____	____	____	6. In checkout lines at the store, may change lines one or more times to another cashier so as to get out of the store more quickly.
7.____	____	____	7. After sleeping a while, may wake up in the early morning hours thinking of the things I have to accomplish, and am unable to go back to sleep again.
8.____	____	____	8. There are times when I rush through my meals in order to get back to work sooner.
9.____	____	____	9. During the work week, when asked to "go out with the boys" to play cards, to fish, to attend a sports event, etc. I am likely to decline.
10.____	____	____	10. Upon retiring for a night's sleep, I, thinking of the days events and the things I have to do, may take an hour or more to fall asleep.

Appendix C *(continued)*

Always or Almost always	Occasionally	Never	
11.____	____	____	11. In a traffic jam, crowd the car in front so as to get the jam moving faster.
12.____	____	____	12. On an elevator, press the "door close" button while waiting for the door to close automatically at a given floor level.
13.____	____	____	13. Almost always have 2 or 3 projects going at the same time.
14.____	____	____	14. Set my morning wake-up alarm almost every night, even on weekends.
15.____	____	____	15. At arising time, after a night's sleep, upon awakening, I am likely to roll over and dose off again.
16.____	____	____	16. If the delivery of a product ordered by mail were delayed being delivered for a considerable length of time, would probably write or call to see what the hang-up was.
17.____	____	____	17. Even though your work on the job was caught up, you'd be inclined to bring some work home, nightly and weekends as well.
18.____	____	____	18. When making a phone call, if the party called, upon answering, asks, "Would you mind holding, I have a call on another line", you you tend to become resentful and impatient.
19.____	____	____	19. Even on vacation, would likely take along job-related materials (books, reports, etc.) to study and review.
20.____	____	____	20. In general, tend to feel guilty when I spend any significant amount of time doing anything except job-related activities.
21.____	____	____	21. Eat breakfast while standing up or pacing about.
22.____	____	____	22. When approaching a red light, and, upon observing that there were no approaching cars in either direction, I would run the light.

Appendix D
Incomplete Sentences

Research Code No.#____

INSTRUCTIONS: You will notice that the sentences below are not complete. We are asking you to make a complete sentence out of each one. You need not be too concerned about grammar or sentence length. Simply write down the first thing that comes into mind. Please work as rapidly as you can, but don't rush, as there is no time limit. If possible, do not omit any. Thanks in advance for your cooperation.

==

1. He worried............
2. One feels useless........
3. I feel................
4. My appetite..............
5. The future............
6. What makes me discouraged.....
7. When rejected, he......
8. My greatest fear.........
9. Morning is............
10. I am.....................
11. Sometimes I want..............
12. Things looked hopeless.....
13. Being with other people........
14. My greatest fault.........
15. What disgusts me most..........
16. I have................
17. I felt like giving up......
18. My sleep..............
19. I still enjoy..............
20. My self-confidence............
21. I.....................
22. One feels needed...........
23. My health.............
24. What makes me angry............
25. My....................
26. One feels guilty...........
27. Life..................
28. If I fail..................
29. If there were no way out.......
30. In the future, I...........
31. What makes me feel "blue" is........
32. I feel inadequate when.........
33. Things looked hopeless when.........
34. Giving up when things look impossible is......
35. Performing below average makes me.........

Appendix D *(continued)*

Research Code No._____

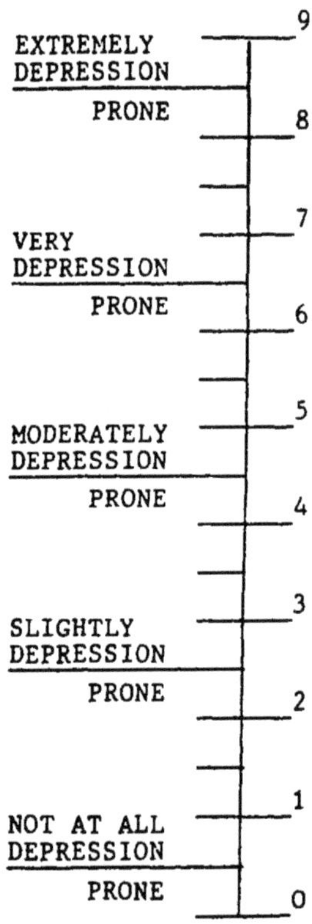

Appendix E
Submariner Frustration Test

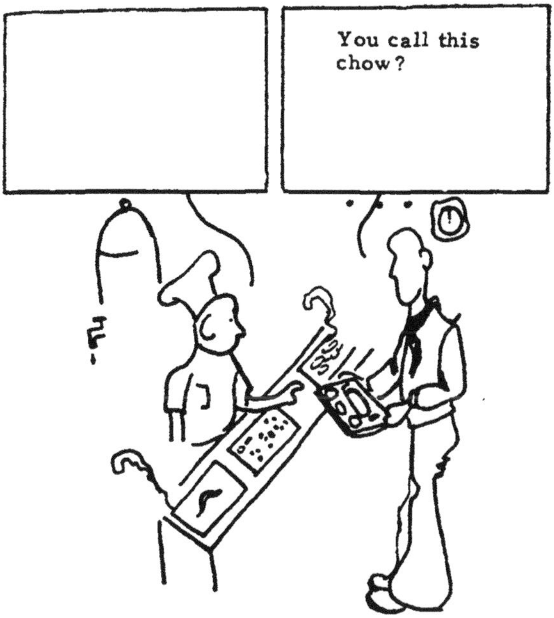
You call this chow?

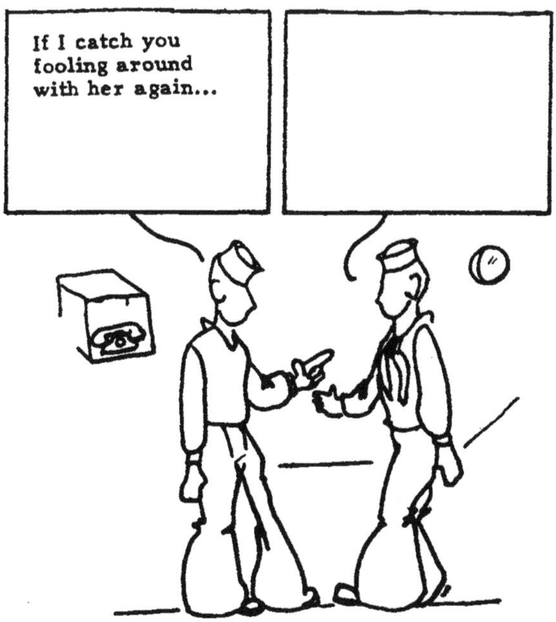
If I catch you fooling around with her again...

Appendix F
Submariner Tell-a-Story Test

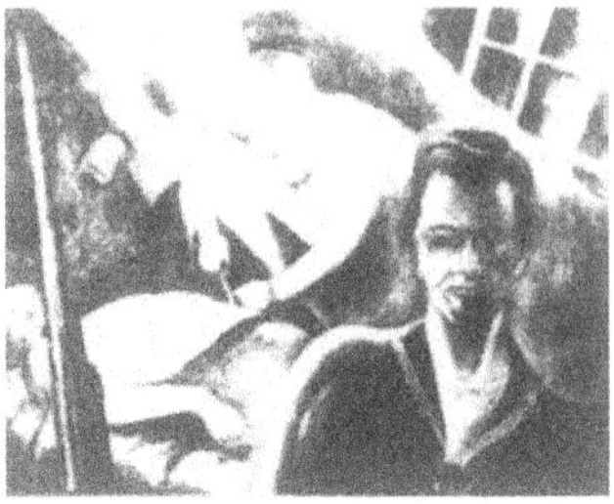

Card I

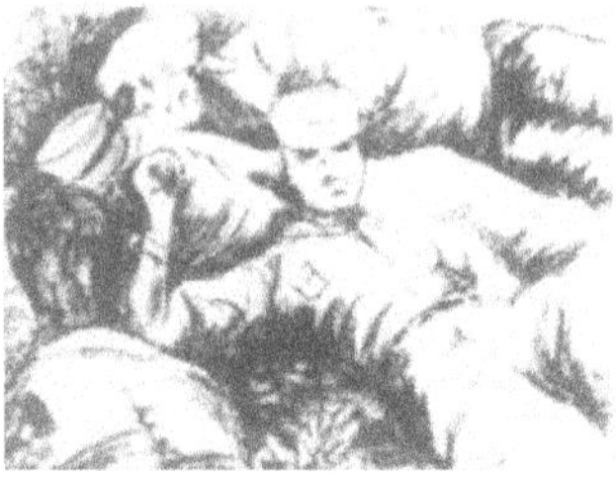

Card II

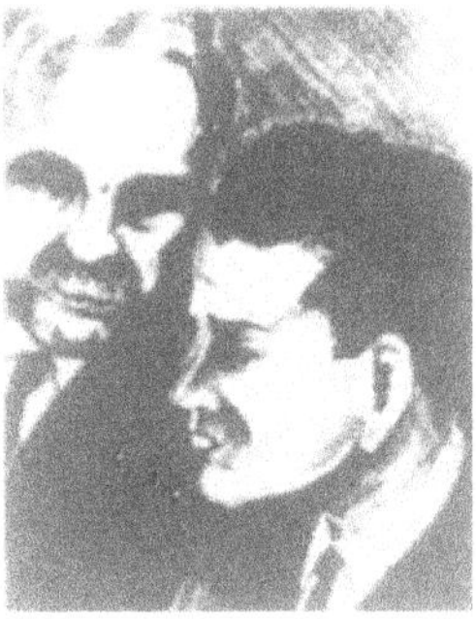

Card III

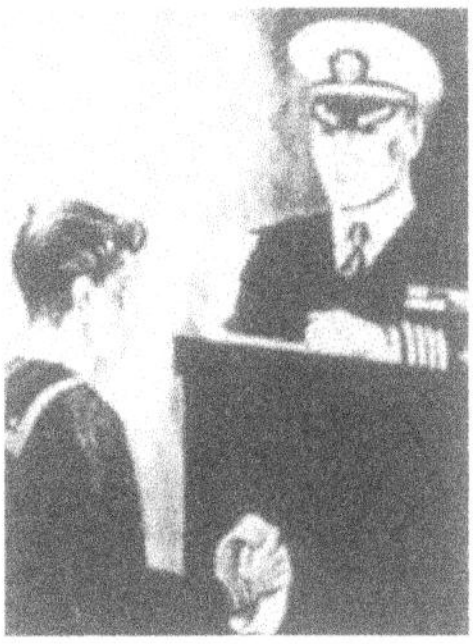

Card IV

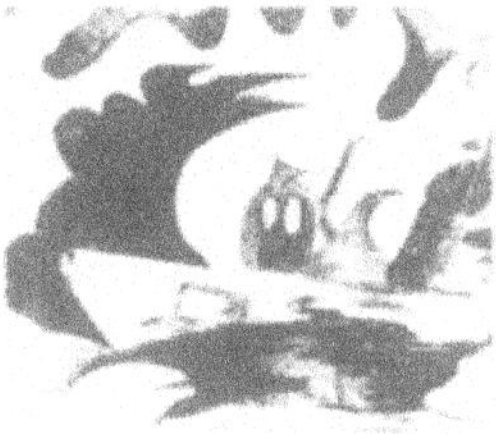

Card V

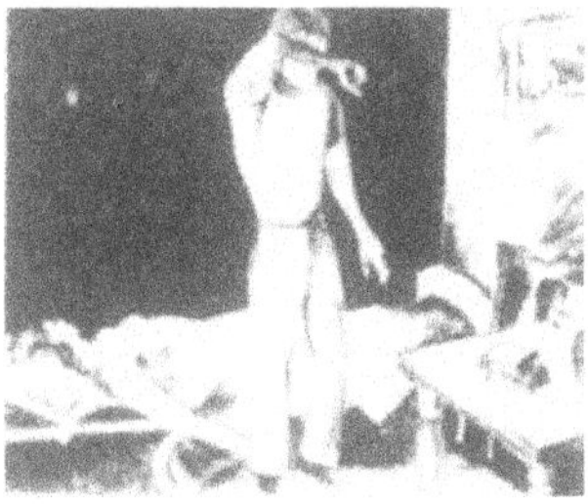

Card VI

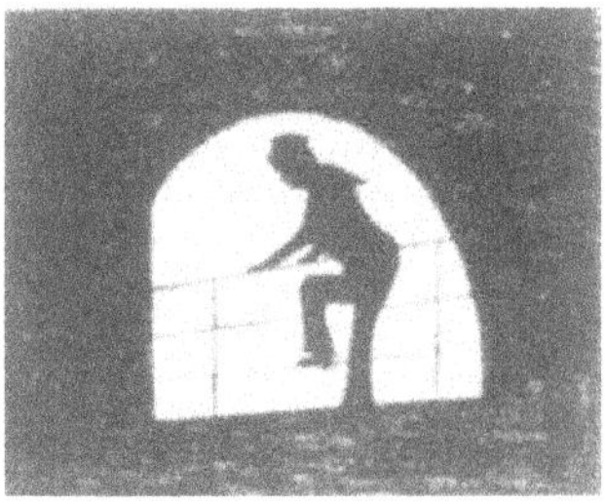

Card VII

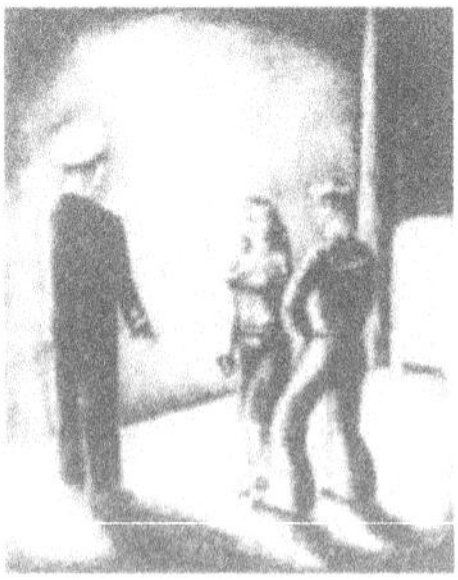

Card VIII

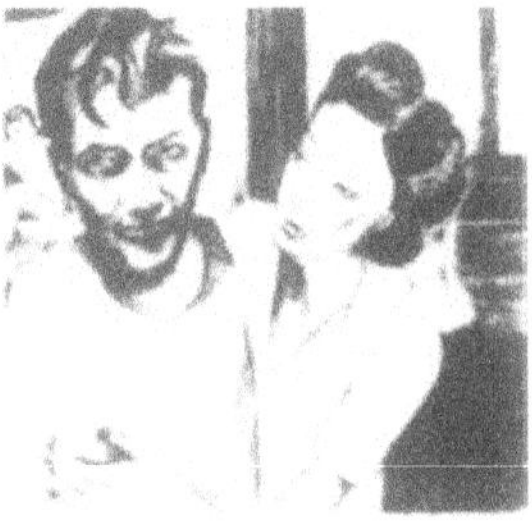

Card IX

Appendix G
Submariner Stereotype Test

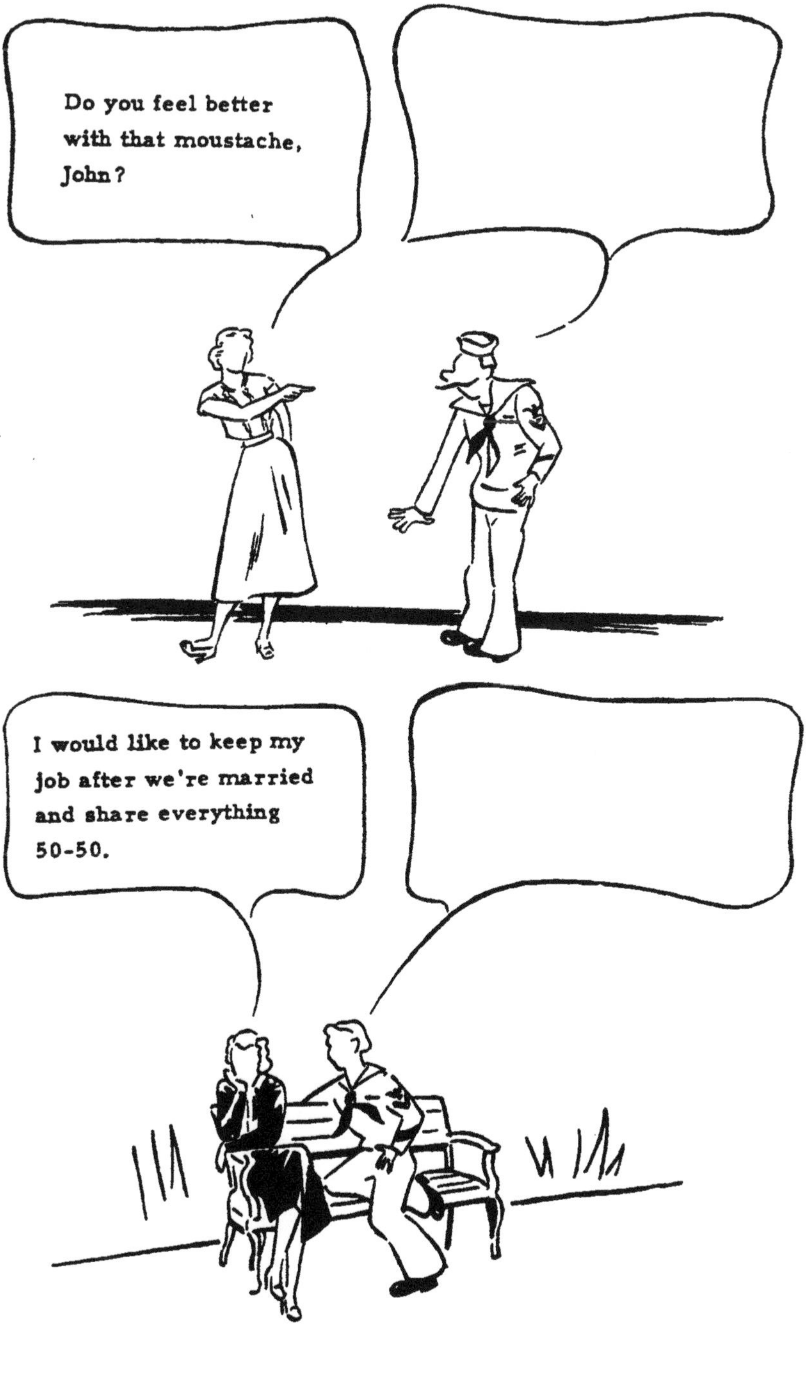
Do you feel better with that moustache, John?
I would like to keep my job after we're married and share everything 50-50.

Appendix H
Submariner Mirth Response Test

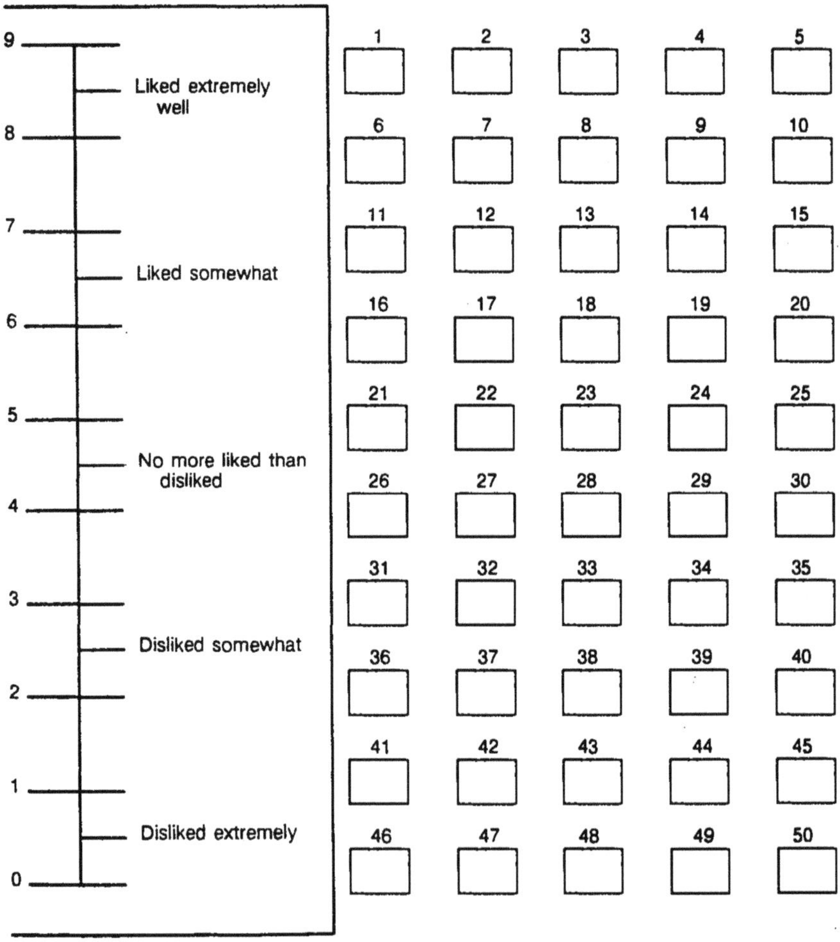

Appendix I
Submariner Attitude Questionnaire

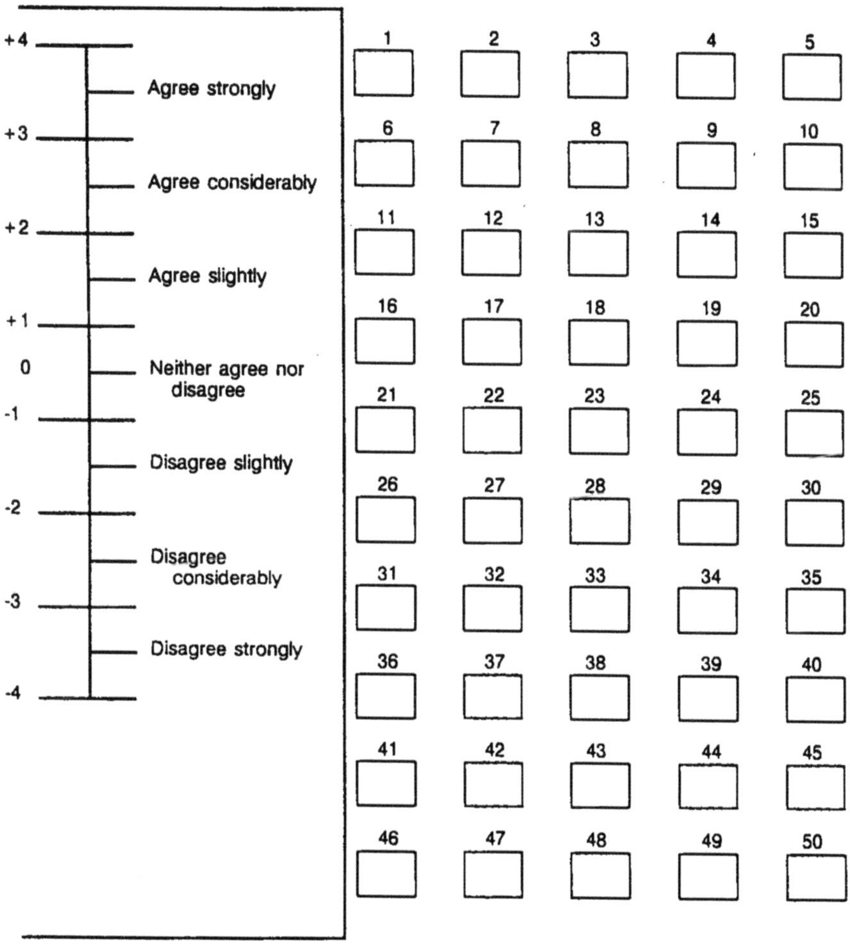

Appendix J
Stress Research Proposal Evaluation Form

Tentative Title of Proposed Research Study: ______________________

Subject Matter Area(s) of the Study: ______________________

Primary Area: ______________________

Secondary Area: ______________________

Probability (Check ✓) Appropriate Point
Percent
0 10 20 30 40 50 60 70 80 90 100

CRITERON CLASS I — Criticality and Focus

A. What is the likelihood that the subject matter area(s) of the proposal contain research problems critical for mission success?

A . . . .
Does not apply ______

B. How likely is it that the central research question(s) or hypotheses can be clearly isolated for study by the present design?

B . . . .
Does not apply ______

C. What is the likelihood that the major research questions, if unanswered, or only partially answered, will significantly reduce mission effectiveness?

C . . . .
Does not apply ______

CRITERON CLASS II — Feasibility

A. What is the likelihood that the appropriate research methodology for the study(ies) either exists or can be developed in a reasonable time span?

A . . . .
Does not apply ______

B. How likely is it that adequate laboratory facilities, instrumentation, computer hardware and software, and qualified professional and support staff can be made available within the funding constraints?

B . . . .
Does not apply ______

C. What is the likelihood that adequate samples of experimental subjects can be made available and that unobtrusive data collection schedules can be implemented?

C . . . .
Does not apply ______

CRITERON CLASS III — Outcomes

A. What is the probability that the research findings will be sufficiently substantive to definitively answer the research question(s) as posed?

A . . . .
Does not apply ______

B. What is the likelihood that some of the findings will provide a meaningful contribution to the scientific community as a whole?

B . . . .
Does not apply ______

C. How likely are the results of the study(ies) to yield significant applied spinoffs useful for the population at large?

C . . . .
Does not apply ______

RATER'S NAME: ______________________

Average Probability: ______________________

Glossary of Stress-Related Terms and Acronyms

AC—affective context, the subjective component of emotions and POSR. Different levels of AC lie on a continuum extending from "pleasant" to "unpleasant."

aerobic exercise—"aerobic," literally, "oxygen in," vigorous physical activity paced so that the blood-oxygen concentration is significantly increased.

allopathic medicine—a medical model based upon the assumption that all diseases have an organic cause or causes. Whereas different diseases may have different causes, nonetheless, all causes are organic in nature.

alpha rhythm—one of the classes of neuroelectrical currents recorded during the EEG, electroencephalographic procedure. "Alpha" occurs with eyes closed during a relaxed but awake state.

ANOVA—analysis of variance, a statistical method for testing the significance of the differences between two or more distributions of data.

ANS—autonomic nervous system, a motor system that controls the functions of the internal organs of the body.

AR—adaptive resources, the total capacity to adapt adequately to the stressors in a specified environment. Approximately equivalent to SCC, or Stress Coping Capacity.

ARC—anticipated reinforcement contingency, a contingency or series of contingencies that have a high probability to be an effective means by which prepotent needs will be satisfied in the *future*.

ARI—Affective Response Inventory, an experimental bipolar scale designed to measure affective response patterns to high-IED situations.

arteriosclerosis—hardening of the arteries, a characteristic of aging.

atherosclerosis—an arterial disease consisting of plaque formation on the walls of the arteries. This condition is thought to be the major cause of hypertension, stroke, and heart attacks.

biofeedback—a behavioral therapeutic technique based upon the Skinnerian learning principle that if a desired instrumental response is reinforced, it tends to be repeated. For example, bioelectronic circuitry produces a "cue" (buzzer) if the desired response (e.g., "heart rate slowing") occurs, but the cue is withheld if the heart rate increases.

CCNW—Co-contingency Network Theory of leadership behavior. *See* Chapter 10.

cholesterol—a member of a class of fats or lipids called sterols. Cholesterol combines with proteins to form HDLP (high-density lipoproteins) or LDLP (low-density lipoproteins), the former described as "good" cholesterol and the latter as "bad" cholesterol. High blood levels of HDLP and low levels of LDLP are believed to contribute to the prevention of heart attack and stroke.

CNS—central nervous system, made up of the brain and spinal cord.

contingency—a dependency, a means to an end for attaining a stated goal or outcome.

Critical Incident Technique—a technique developed by John Flannagan for delineating important task elements of a specific job from descriptive anecdotes related by expert incumbents in that particular job.

diathesis model—a medical model that makes the assumption that every disease process, including POSR, has a biogenetic or organic cause.

distress—or dystress, literally, maladaptive stress (i.e., POSR) with intensity sufficiently high to cause decompensatory processes, operationally defined by subjective or affective symptomatology.

EDC—electrodermal conductance, recordings of the bioelectric conductance of the skin, which, in the palm of the hand, for example, is enervated by the SNS, but uniquely involves cholinergic (releases acetylcholine at the synapses) rather than adrenergic (releases adrenaline at the synapses) nerve fibers.

EEG—electroencephalogram, the so-called brain wave tracing, consists of a graphic recording of the bioelectric current produced by the billions of neurons in the brain.

EMG—electromyogram, a graphic record of the electric currents originating from muscle tissue.

endorphin—a morphine-like neurohormone found in the brain. It is thought to be related to depression and other affective disorders.

epinephrine—same as adrenaline and is a neurotransmitter secreted by the adrenal medulla. It is found in most of the post-ganglionic fibers of the SNS. It acts as a stimulant to the SNS.

eustress—adaptable or "good" stress. Coined by Hans Selye, the term "eustress" refers to a stress reaction (POSR) of intensity sufficiently low so that compensatory mechanisms are adequate to sustain homeostasis.

expectancy—the subjective probability that a specific contingency or combination of contingencies will result in goal attainment.

FBM—Fleet Ballistic Missile submarine, a nuclear-powered, single reactor "sub" that is armed with nuclear warhead missiles.

ganglion—a cluster of neurons and nerve fibers located outside of the brain and spinal cord.

GAS—General Adaptation Syndrome, a concept developed by Hans Selye to explain the three phases of a stress reaction: alarm, resistance, and exhaustion.

glycogenesis—the processes involved in the synthesis of glycogen (sugar) in the liver.

glycogenolysis—the processes by which glycogen, a carbohydrate, is broken down in the liver.

GTPSS—Global Trait Psychological Screening System, a set of rating scales developed by the U.S. Naval submarine service to assess the qualifications of the recruits for the nuclear submarine service.

homeostasis—literally, homo- "same," stasis, "state," that is, any process by which conditions within the body are maintained relatively constant, for example, the acid-base balance or pH of the blood.

hypersphere—a geometric, multidimensional sphere, imaginary in the mathematical sense, into which the vectorially represented tests or other measures involved in factor analyses are projected.

IED—intensity of environmental demands, the numerator of the basic equation for POSR in this text (i.e., POSR = K [IED/AR]). IED may be calculated by summing the SEP's of the stressors identified within the environmental context of concern.

IVP—intervention procedure. Any technique or procedure aimed at reducing the intensity level of POSR—for examples, *see* Table 8.2.

LB—leadership behavior, certain behavior or activity of a person or persons that influences the behavior of the members of a specified group.

LIV—Law of Initial Value, a statistical principle asserting that prestress or baseline measures tend to be negatively correlated with change-scores (poststress-prestress scores) for the same measure [158].

locus of control—a conceptual theory that dichotomizes personalities into "internalizers," who assume that life events are under their own control, and "externalizers," who assume that these events are controlled by causal processes outside themselves.

MEL—minimum effective level, the most appropriate level (individual, group, intergroup, or organizational) to apply an IVP(s) aimed at reducing the intensity level of POSR.

micromhos—a measure of electrical conductance used in experiments involving the GSR (galvanic skin response) and EDC (electrodermal conductance).

moderator variables—or "mods," are variables that systematically affect the correlation between two or more other variables. For example, IQ test scores are a "mod" for the correlation between SAT scores and the grade point average of college students. In the ABC model, "mods" (age or gender, for instance) affect the relationship between POSR and the IED/AR ratio in Equation 4.1.

MPTRP—Myoperceptual Tension Reduction Procedure, a modification of the Jacobson Progressive Relaxation Technique to include a classical conditioning adjunct.

nerve tract—a collection or bundle of nerve fibers having the same origin, function, and termination.

neuroleptic drug—a family of nonsedating drugs, including tranquilizers, that are used to control the anxiety component of POSR. Other labels for this group of substances are psychoactive or psychotropic classes of drugs.

neurotransmitters—any substance that changes the rate of neural transmission at the synapses. Dopamine and norepinephrine are examples of these substances.

NPP—Need Prepotency Profile (Pattern), the relative strength or prepotency (capacity to control behavior) of a given set of needs functioning at a particular time.

operational definition—a concept, process, or phenomena defined in terms of the technique or method by which it is measured (for instance, intelligence is measured by an IQ test, which is an operational definition of the term).

OR—outcome ratio, same as expectancy ratio and refers to the expectancy (subjective probability) of the ratio of reinforcement to punishment, or $RF^{\pm}/Pu^{\pm}$. OR is usually expressed in percentages.

PAQ—Personal Attitude Questionnaire, an experimental attitude scale designed to identify submariner recruits with militantly pacifistic attitudes.

personality—the unique pattern of traits, either structural or functional, that describes an individual's singular style of adjustment to life.

phi coefficient—a correlation statistic used with nominal scale data.

PNS—parasympathetic nervous system, a branch of the autonomic nervous system (ANS). See Tables 3.1 and 3.2.

POSR—patterns of stress reactivity, used in this text as an equivalent to the term *stress*. POSR includes six classes of psychophysiological processes. *See* Figure 3.1 and Table 3.3.

PPM—psychiatric plimsoll mark, "plimsoll mark" literally is a nautical term referring to the line on the side of a cargo ship, not to be exceeded by the water line when the ship is fully loaded. Analogously, PPM is a "breaking point," an index of the intensity of POSR above which decompensatory symptoms are likely to occur. PPM was proposed by G. L. Freeman[38].

PRC—perceived reinforcement contingency, perception or identification of a mode-to-goal, an algorithm in computer language, or, in Skinnerian terms, an instrumental behavior with an estimable expectancy to result in goal attainment.

progressive relaxation—a technique for reducing muscular tension developed by E. Jacobson. It is similar to MPTRP (Myoperceptual Tension Reduction Procedure).

psychosomatic medicine—the branch of medicine that assumes that the "psyche" or mind, more specifically, emotions, affect the structural and functional characteristics of organ systems, the "soma."

Pu—punishment. Pu may be positive (Pu+), withholding positive reinforcement, or negative (Pu−), causing an unpleasant outcome (−AC), following the implementation of a given contingency.

Q-card—a 3 × 5 or other size file card upon which descriptors (traits, mood states, and so on) are written. Q-cards are employed in Q-sorts such as used in SIRO (Stressor Identification and Rank Ordering) procedure.

Q-sort—with behavioral statements, personality traits, or specific environmental stressors written on Q-cards, a rank order distribution of these cards is developed according to an instructional set, for example, from most to least characteristic, or, in SIRO, sort the stressors (on Q-cards) from high to low SEP.

RBD—rubber band demonstration, a classroom procedure for explaining the ABC model of stress.

RC—reinforcement contingency, behavior or a sequence of goal-directed behaviors leading to, or upon which, a specified outcome or consequence is dependent.

RF—reinforcement. RF may be positive (RF+) if the contingency results in AC+, and negative (RF−) if the contingency allows for avoidance of −AC, or negative punishment, Pu−.

Rumpelstiltskin Fallacy—the fallacy that the very act of naming or labeling a phenomenon or event explains the cause of that phenomenon or event—based upon a children's nineteenth-century fairy tale by the Grimm brothers of Germany.

SAD_{50}—significant adaptive decrement in 50 percent of a given population sample. SAD_{50} is analogous to LD_{50}, an index used in pharmacology to indicate the dosage of a specific drug or other agent that is lethal for 50 percent of a test sample of animals.

SCC—stress coping capacity, an index purported to measure individual differences in a person's ability to adapt adequately to a specified set of stressors.

SCS—stress coping strategy, any systematic attempt to remove or mitigate the intensity level of POSR.

SD—standard deviation, a statistical measure of score variation within a score distribution[36].

SEM—standard error of measurement, a statistic that yields an estimate of the reliability of an individual's score on a specified test or other measure.

SEP—stress evocation potential, a measure of a specific stressor's probability to produce significant POSR for a person or persons exposed to that stressor.

serotonin—a neurohormone similar to adrenalin but much more powerful. It is found in the brain, intestines, and blood platelets. The concentration level in the blood is thought to be complexly related to some depressive disorders and possibly schizophrenia.

SIRO—stressor identification and rank ordering, a procedure for Q-sorting stressors (written on Q-cards) according to their SEP (stress evocation potential).

SIRT—stressor identification and ranking therapy, therapeutic techniques applied to the high-SEP stressors delineated by SIRO.

SNS—sympathetic nervous system, a branch of the autonomic nervous system or ANS. Sometimes called the adrenergic system.

somatopsychic causation—the opposite causal direction from psychosomatic, that is, the functional and structural characteristic of organ systems directly affect emotional reactivity (POSR).

stress—by common dictionary definition, "a condition of extreme mental tension"[126]. In this book, however, POSR is used as the equivalent of the term *stress*. POSR consist of six classes of processes such as ANS, CNS, skeletal musculature, and so on (*see* Figure 3.1 and Table 3.3). POSR are typically concomitants of negative emotions (fear, anxiety, and panic for example). POSR occur in an environmental situation in which the IED "Intensity of Environmental Demands) significantly exceeds the person's AR (adaptive resources) (*see* Equation 4.1).

stressors—environmental impediments or barriers to goal-directed behavior. It is assumed that these blockages evoke acute or chronic negative emotions, such as anxiety, fear, panic, tremors, and so on. The sum total of this emotional reactivity is labeled *stress*, or more appropriately POSR (Patterns of Stress Reactivity).

synapses—regions of contact between the axons and dendrites of two or more adjacent neurons.

TMS—Temporomandibular syndrome, a tension condition in the temporal and mandibular muscles of the jaw. TMS is often treated by biofeedback.

topological psychology—literally, topo-, space or place—a field theoretical approach developed by Kurt Lewin. The theory assumes that behavior, represented by vectors, occurs within a topological space or field. Like an amoeba, this space for a given person is invariant in total area, but may bend, stretch, contort, and otherwise transform into an infinite number of forms.

triglycerides—fatty substances similar to cholesterol found in the blood. They are thought to be a contributing factor in atherosclerosis.

TRS—tension reduced state, the level of reduction in muscular tension reached at each phase of the MPTRP (Myoperceptual Tension Reduction Procedure).

tryptophan—an amino acid found in proteins from which it is released during digestion of food. Its concentration in the blood appears to be correlated in some complex manner with food metabolism.

T-scores—sometimes called McCall scores, are normalized, area-transformed scores yielding a normal distribution with a mean of fifty and a standard deviation of ten T-score units.

valence—a term borrowed from chemistry by Kurt Lewin. It refers to the polarity (plus or minus), affinity, or "value" of a goal or satisfier within a force field. Valences of goals affect the alignment of motivational vectors in that field.

variance—a statistic indicating the amount of variation of scores within a distribution.

work stressors—stressors typically found in the work place. Examples of work stressors are noise, glare, heat, cold, interpersonal tension, and work overload and underload.

X—mathematical symbol for the independent or manipulated variable in the linear equation representing the scientific method, $Y = f(X)$.

Y—mathematical symbol for the dependent or experimental variable in scientific experimentation. For example, *Y* represents changes in the emotional and behavioral components of POSR resulting from some systematic changes in the IED (the *X*'s in the experiment) in typical stress studies.

z-score—or standard deviation score, is calculated by subtracting each raw score from the arithmetical mean of the score distribution and dividing that remainder by the standard deviation. A distribution of z-scores has a mean of "0" and a standard deviation of "1," which is the basis for calling this distribution the "unit normal curve."

Z-score—a linear transformation of the z-score obtained by the formula, Z-score = 10z + 50. The distribution of Z-scores has, therefore, a mean of fifty and an SD of ten Z-score units. Z-scores equal T-scores only in distributions that precisely fit the equation of the normal or Gaussian curve.

References

The following references are listed both alphabetically and numerically. They are referred to in the text by number.

1. Alderfer, C. P. *Existence, relatedness and growth: Human needs in organizational settings*. New York: Free Press, 1972.
2. Aldrich, H., and Herker, D. Boundary spanning roles and organizational structure. *Academy of Management Review, 2, 1977*, 217–30.
3. Allport, G. W. *The nature of personality*. Reading, MA.: Addison-Wesley, 1950.
4. Ax, A. F. The physiological differentiation between fear and anger in humans. *Psychosomatic Medicine, 15, 1953*, 433–42.
5. Bandura, A. *Principles of behavior modification*. New York: Holt, 1969.
6. Barrios, A. A. *Toward greater freedom and happiness*. Knoxville, TN.: S.P.C. Press, 1962.
7. Barron, F., and Harrington, D. M. Creativity, intelligence, and personality. *Annual Review of Psychology, 32, 1981*, 439–76.
8. Basowitz, H., Persky, H., Korchin, S., and Grinker, R. *Anxiety and stress*. New York: McGraw-Hill, 1955.
9. Bass, B. M. The leaderless group discussion. *Psychological Bulletin, 51, 1954*, 465–92.
10. Bavelas, A. Communication patterns in task-oriented groups. *Journal of the Acoustical Society of America, 22, 1950*, 725–30.
11. Benne, K., and Sheats, P. Functional roles of group members. *Journal of Social Issues, 2, 1948*, 42–47.
12. Berger, H. Ueber das elektrenkepalogramm des menschen I. *Archives Psychiat. Nervenker, 87, 1929*, 527–70.
13. Bergin, A. E. Some implications of psychotherapy research for therapeutic practice. *Journal of Abnormal Psychology, 71, 1966*, 235–46.
14. Berne, E. *Transactional analysis in psychotherapy*. New York: Grove Press, 1961.

15. Berstein, D. A., and Borkovec, T. D. *Progressive relaxation training: A manual for the helping professions*. Champaign, IL: Research Press, 1973.
16. Blake, R. R., and Mouton, J. R. *The new managerial grid*. Houston, TX: Gulf, 1978.
17. Blanchard, E. B., and Epstein, L. H. *A biofeedback primer*. Reading, MA: Addison-Wesley, 1978.
18. Bowers, K. S. *Hypnosis for the seriously curious*. Monterey, CA: Brooks/Cole, 1976.
19. Bridges, K. B. Emotional development in early infancy. *Child Development, 3, 1932*, 324–41.
20. Brief, A. P., Schuler, R. S., and Van Sell, M. *Managing job stress*. Boston: Little, Brown and Co., 1981.
21. Cannon, W. B. Stresses and the strains of homeostasis. *American Journal of Medical Science, 189, 1935*, 1–14.
22. Cattell, R. B. *The description and measurement of personality*. New York: World Book Co., 1946.
23. Cattell, R. B., and Luborsky, L. B. P-technique demonstrated as a new clinical method for determining personality and symptom structure. *Journal of General Psychology, 42, 1950*, 3–24.
24. Chan, K. B. Individual differences in reactions to stress and their personality and situational determinants. *Social Science and Medicine, 11, 1977*, 89–103.
25. Cooper, C. L., and Payne, R. *Stress at work*. New York: John Wiley and Sons, 1978.
26. Cox, T. *Stress*. Baltimore: University Park Press, 1978.
27. Crissy, W. J. E., and Pashalian, S. Aids to the interview: The submariner stereotype. *U.S. Naval Submarine Medical Research Lab. Report No. 214*, 1952.
28. Detre, T. P., and Jarecki, H. G. *Modern psychiatric treatment*. Philadelphia: J.B. Lippincott Co., 1971.
29. *Diagnostic and Statistical Manual of Mental Disorders (DSM-III-R)*, American Psychiatric Association. Washington, D.C., 1987.
30. Dohrenwend, B. P., and Shrout, P. E. "Hassles" in the conceptualization and measurement of life stress variables. *American Psychologist, 41, 1986*, 780–85.
31. Dollard, J., and Miller, N. *Frustration and aggression*. New Haven: Yale University Press, 1939.
32. Edwards, M. How does stress affect nutrition? *Nutrition Quarterly, 11(1), 1987*, 3–7.
33. Ellis, A. *Reason and emotion in psychotherapy*. New York: Lyle Stuart, 1962.
34. Ellis, A., and Harper, R. A. *A guide to rational living*. New York: Lyle Stuart, 1968.
35. Fiedler, F. E. *A theory of leadership effectiveness*. New York: McGraw-Hill, 1967.
36. Fisher, R. A. *Statistical methods for research workers*. Edinburgh: Oliver and Boyd, 1925.
37. Foster, R. J., and Carnaghan, J. G. Prediction of submarine school success through the use of selected themes in the Navy Thematic Apperception test. *U.S. Naval Submarine Medical Research Lab. Report No. 263*, 1955.
38. Freeman, G. L. *The energetics of human behavior*. Ithaca, NY: Cornell University Press, 1948.

39. Freeman, G. L., Manson, G., Katzoff, E. T., and Pathman, J. H. The stress interview. *Journal of Abnormal and Social Psychology, 37, 1942*, 427–47.
40. Friedman, M., and Roseman, R. H. *Type A behavior and your heart*. Greenwich, CT: Fawcett Press, 1974.
41. Fruchter, B. *Introduction to factor analysis*. New York: D. Van Nostrand Co., 1954.
42. Fuller, G. D. Current status of biofeedback in clinical practice. *American Psychologist, 33, 1978*, 39–48.
43. Funkenstein, D. H., King, S. H., and Drolette, M. E. *Mastery of stress*. Cambridge, MA: Harvard University Press, 1957.
44. Gengerelli, J. A., and Kirkner, F. J. *The psychological variables in human cancer*. Los Angeles: University of California Press, 1954.
45. Golembiewski, R. T. The laboratory approach to organizational change: Schema of a method. *Public Administration Review, 27, 1967*, 211–15.
46. Gross, E. The definition of organizational goals. *British Journal of Sociology, 20, 1969*. 277–94.
47. Guilford, J. P. *Personality*. New York: McGraw-Hill, 1959.
48. Harms, E. The development of humor. *Journal of Abnormal and Social Psychology, 38, 1943*, 351–69.
49. Hartmann, E. L. *The functions of sleep*. New Haven: Yale University Press, 1973.
50. Heider, F. *The psychology of interpersonal relations*. New York: Wiley, 1958.
51. Helms, D. B., and Turner, J. S. *Exploring child behavior*. Philadelphia: W.B. Saunders Co., 1976.
52. Hinkle, L. E. Occupation, education and coronary heart disease. *Science, 161, 1968*, 238–46.
53. Holmes, T. H., and Rahe, R. H. The social readjustment rating scale. *Journal of Psychosomatic Medicine, 11, 1967*, 213–18.
54. Homme, L. E. Perspectives in psychology, XXIV. Control of coverants, the operants of the mind. *Psychological Record, 15, 1965*, 501–11.
55. House, R. J. A path-goal theory of leader effectiveness. *Administrative Science Quarterly, 16, 1971*, 321–38.
56. Ivancevich, J. M., and Matteson, M. *Stress and work: A managerial perspective*. Glenview, IL: Scott, Foresman and Co., 1980.
57. Jacobson, E. *Progressive relaxation*. Chicago: University Press, 1938.
58. Janis, I. *Victims of groupthink: A psychological study of foreign policy decisions and fiascos*. New York: Houghton-Mifflin, 1972.
59. Jepsen, D. A. Occupational decision development over the high school years. *Journal of Vocational Behavior, 7, 1975*, 225–37.
60. Kamiya, J. Conscious control of brainwaves. *Psychology Today, 1, 1968*, 56–60.
61. Kasl, S., and Cobb, S. Blood pressure changes in men undergoing job loss: A preliminary report. *Psychosomatic Medicine, 32, 1970*, 19–38.
62. King, B. T. Some correlates of disqualification in the submarine service. *U.S.N. Submarine Medical Research Laboratory Report No. 291*, 1957.
63. Kotter, J. P. Power, dependence and effective management. *Harvard Business Review, 55, 1977*, 135–36.
64. Krech, D., and Crutchfield, S. *Theory and problems of social psychology*. New York: McGraw-Hill, 1948.

65. Kroger, W. S., and Fezler, W. D. *Hypnosis and behavior modification: Imagery conditioning*. Philadelphia: J.B. Lippincott, 1976.
66. Lacey, J. I., and Lacey, B. The law of initial value in the longitudinal study of autonomic constitution: reproducibility of autonomic responses and response patterns over a four-year interval. *Annals of the New York Academy of Sciences, 98, 1962*, 1257–90.
67. Lazarus, R. S., DeLongis, A., Folkman, S., and Gruen, R. Stress and adaptational outcomes: The problem of confounded measures. *American Psychologist, 40, 1985*, 770–79.
68. Lewin, K. *Principles of topological psychology*. New York: McGraw-Hill, 1936.
69. Lewin, K. Time perspective and morale. In C. Watson (Ed.). *Civilian morale*. Boston: Houghton Mifflin, 1942, pp. 48–70.
70. Lewin, K. *Field theory in social science*. New York: Harper and Row, 1951.
71. Lewinson, D. J. The mid-life transition: A period in adult psychological development. *Psychiatry, 40, 1977*, 99–112.
72. Liebowitz, C. To release stress—exercise! *New York State Dental Journal, May, 1989*, 36–37.
73. Linstone, H. A., and Turoff, M. (Eds.) *The Delphi methods: Techniques and applications*. Reading, MA: Addison-Wesley, 1975.
74. Lock, E. A., Shaw, K. N., Saari, L. M., and Latham, G. P. Goal setting and task performance. *Psychological Bulletin, 90, 1981*, 125–52.
75. Lowenthal, M. F., Thurnher, M., and Chiriboga, D. *Four stages of life*. San Francisco: Jossey-Bass, 1975.
76. MacKinnon, D. W. The nature and nurture of creative talent. *American Psychologist, 17, 1962*, 484–95.
77. Maslow, A. H. A theory of human motivation. *Psychological Review, 50, 1943*, 370–96.
78. McClelland, D. C. *The achieving society*. Princeton, NJ: Van Nostrand Reinhold Co., 1961.
79. McClelland, D. C., and Burnham, D. H. Power driven managers: Good guys make bum bosses. *Psychology Today*, December 1975.
80. McClelland, D. C. *The achievement motive*. New York: Appleton-Century Crofts, 1953.
81. McGrath, J. E. Stress and behavior in organizations. In M. D. Dunnette (Ed.). *Handbook of Industrial and Organizational Psychology*. Chicago: Rand McNally and Co., 1976, 1351–95.
82. Meehl, P. E. *Clinical vs. statistical prediction*. Minneapolis: University of Minnesota Press, 1954.
83. Melton, A. W. (Ed.) *Apparatus tests*. Washington, D.C.: Government Printing Office, 1947.
84. Miller, D., and Form, W. *Industrial sociology*. New York: Harper and Row, 1951.
85. Moses, J., Steptoe, A., Mathews, A., and Edwards, S. The effects of exercise training on mental well-being in the normal population: A controlled trial. *Journal of Psychosomatic Research, 33 (No. 1), 1989*, 47–60.
86. Mueller, E. F. Psychological and physiological correlates of work overload among university professors. Doctoral dissertation, University of Michigan, Ann Arbor, 1965.
87. Muenzinger, K. *The science of behavior*. New York: Harper, 1942.

88. Murray, H. A., and Morgan, C. D. *Explorations in personality*. New York: Oxford Book Co., 1938.

89. Nadel, S. F. *The foundations of social anthropology*. New York: Cohen and West, 1951.

90. Nadler, D. A. *Feedback and organization development: Using data-based methods*. Reading, MA: Addison-Wesley, 1977.

91. Phares, E. J. Differential utilization of information as a function of internal-external control. *Journal of Personality, 36, 1968*, 649–62.

92. Pyle, R. Corporate fitness programs—How do they shape up. *AMACON, 1979*, 58–67.

93. Rimm, D. C., and Masters, J. C. *Behavioral theory: Techniques and empirical findings*. New York: Academic Press, 1974.

94. Roberts, M., and Harris, G. T. Wellness at work. *Psychology Today, May 1989*, 54–58.

95. Rosenzweig, S. *Aggressive behavior and the Rosenzweig Picture Frustration Study*. New York: Praeger, 1978.

96. Ruesch, J., and Brodsky, C. M. Concept of social disability. *Archives of General Psychiatry, 19, 1968*, 394–403.

97. Salter, A. *Conditioned reflex therapy*. New York: Farrar, Straus, 1949.

98. Saunders, D. R. Moderator variables in prediction. *Educational Psychological Measurement, 16, 1956*, 209–22.

99. Schuler, R. S. Time management: A stress management technique. *Personnel Journal, 58, 1979*, 851–54.

100. Schultz, J. H., and Luthe, W. *Autogenic Training*. New York: Grune and Stratton, 1959.

101. Schwartz, I., and Sandberg, N. E. The effect of time in the submarine service on vision. *U.S. Naval Submarine Medical Research Lab Report No. 253*, 1954.

102. Schwartz, G. E., Shapiro, D., and Tursky, B. Learned control of cardiovascular integration in man through operant conditioning. *Psychosomatic Medicine, 33, 1971*, 57

103. Scott, E. L. Perceptions of organizations and leadership behavior: A study of perceptions of organization structure and their social correlates in a submarine squadron of the U.S. Navy. *ONR Contract N6ori–17 T.O. II N.R. 171, 123, Ohio State University*, Columbus, Ohio, 1949.

104. Scott, W. A. Research definitions of mental health and mental illness. *Psychological Bulletin, 55, 1958*, 29–45.

105. Selye, H. *The stress of life*. New York: McGraw-Hill, 1976.

106. Selye, H. *Stress*. Montreal: Acta, 1950.

107. Selye, H. Confusion and controversy in the stress field. *Journal of Human Stress, 1, 1975*, 37–44.

108. Skeat, W. W. *A concise etymological dictionary of the English language*. Oxford: Oxford University Press, 1958.

109. Sloane, R. B., et al. *Psychotherapy versus behavior therapy*. Cambridge, MA: Harvard University Press, 1975.

110. Smeltzer, L. R., and Kedia, B. L. Knowing the ropes: Organizational requirements for quality circles. *Business Horizons, 28, 1985*, 30–34.

111. Smith, B. M. *The polygraph in contemporary psychology*. San Francisco: Freeman, 1971.

112. Solomon, R. L. Punishment. *American Psychologist, 19, 1964*, 239–53.
113. Solomon, R. L., and Wynne, L. C. Traumatic avoidance learning acquisition in normal dogs. *Psychological Monographs, (Whole No. 54), 57*, 1953.
114. Stephenson, W. *The study of behavior: Q-technique and its methodology*. Chicago: University of Chicago Press, 1953.
115. Terman, L. M. *Genetic studies of genius*. Palo Alto, CA: Stanford University Press, 1925.
116. Thomas, K. W. Conflict and conflict management. In M. D. Dunette (Ed.). *Handbook of industrial and organizational psychology*. Chicago: Rand McNally, 1976, pp. 889–935.
117. Thorndike, E. L. *The psychology of learning*. New York: Teachers College, Columbia University Press, 1921.
118. Thurstone, L. L. *Multiple factor analysis*. Chicago: University of Chicago Press, 1947.
119. Thurstone, L. L. *Vectors of the mind*. Chicago: University of Chicago Press, 1935.
120. Thurstone, L. L. *Creative talent: Proceedings of the 1950 invitational conference on testing problems*. Princeton, NJ: Educational Testing Service, 1951.
121. Thurstone, L. L., and Degan, J. W. A factorial study of the Supreme Court. *Psychometric Laboratory Report No. 64, University of Chicago*, 7 pp.
122. Torrance, E. P. Leadership in the survival of small isolated groups. In *Symposium in preventive and social psychiatry*. Washington, D.C.: Walter Reed Army Institute of Research, 1957, pp. 309–27.
123. U.S. Department of Defense (DOD). *Game without winners: A basic handbook for commanders, DOD Directive Gen–33, July 19, 1968*.
124. Van de Ven, A. H., Delbecq, A. L., and Koenig, R., Jr. Determinants of coordination modes within organizations. *American Sociological Review, 41, 1976*, 322–38.
125. Wallace, R. K. Physiological effects of transcendental meditation. *Science, 167, 1970*, 1951.
126. Warren, H. C. *Dictionary of psychology*. New York: Houghton Mifflin Co., 1934.
127. Weitz, J., and Adler, S. The optimal use of simulation. *Journal of Applied Psychology, 58(2), 1973*, 219–24.
128. Wenger, M. A. Studies of autonomic balance in the Army Air Forces personnel. *Comparative Psychology Monograph, 19, 1948*, 1–111.
129. Weybrew, B. B. Q-methodology in criterion research. *U.S.N. Submarine Medical Research Laboratory Report No. 239*, 1953.
130. Weybrew, B. B. Predicting the adjustment to long periods of confinement: A study of factor analytic methodology. Doctoral dissertation, University of Colorado, Boulder, 1955.
131. Weybrew, B. B. Psychological and psychophysiological effects of long periods of submergence I. Analysis of data collected during a 265-hour habitability cruise of the USS Nautilus. *U.S.N. Submarine Medical Research Laboratory Report No. 281*, 1957.
132. Weybrew, B. B. Patterns of reaction to stress as revealed by a factor analysis of autonomic-change measures and behavioral observations. *Journal of General Psychology, 60, 1959*, 253–64.
133. Weybrew, B. B. Behavioral energetics: A factor analytical study of individual

differences in modes of energy discharge resulting from experimentally-induced frustration. *U.S.N. Submarine Medical Research Laboratory Report No. 378*, 1962.

134. Weybrew, B. B. Prediction of adjustment to long submergence aboard a fleet ballistic missile submarine I. Interrelationship of the adjustment criteria. *U.S.N. Submarine Medical Research Laboratory Report No. 383*, 1962.

135. Weybrew, B. B. Accuracy of time estimation and muscular tension. *Perceptual and Motor Skills, 17, 1963*, 118.

136. Weybrew, B. B. Psychological problems of prolonged periods of marine submergence. In Burns, N. M., Chambers, R. M., and Hendler, E. (Eds.). *Unusual environments and human behavior*. New York: Collier-Macmillan, 1963, pp. 85–125.

137. Weybrew, B. B. Selection of men for hazardous duty from indices of autonomic nervous system reactivity. *U.S.N. Submarine Medical Research Laboratory Memorandum Report No. 65–1*, 1965.

138. Weybrew, B. B. Patterns of psychophysiological response to military stress. In Appley, M. H. and Trumbull, R. (Eds.). *Psychological stress: Issues in research*. New York: Appleton-Century-Crofts, 1966, pp. 324–54.

139. Weybrew, B. B. Characteristics of the submarine line officer: A factor analytical study of the candidate for the nuclear submarine service. *U.S.N. Submarine Medical Research Laboratory Report No. 616*, 1970.

140. Weybrew, B. B. Submarine crew effectiveness during submerged missions of sixty or more days duration. *U.S.N. Submarine Medical Research Laboratory Report No. 686*, 1971.

141. Weybrew, B. B. Diver adaptability during a nitrox saturation dive at 7 ATA. *Undersea Biomedical Research, 5 (No. 3), 1978*, 259–73.

142. Weybrew, B. B. The Zeigarnik phenomenon revisited: Implications for enhancement of morale. *Perceptual and Motor Skills, 58, 1985*, 223–26.

143. Weybrew, B. B. Psychologic screening of job applicants. *Seminars in Occupational Medicine, 1(2), June 1986*, 141–51.

144. Weybrew, B. B. Prediction of adjustment to long submergence aboard an FBM submarine IV: Psychophysiological indices. *U.S.N. Submarine Medical Research Laboratory Report No. 416*, 1964.

145. Weybrew, B. B. Three decades of nuclear submarine research: Implications for space and antarctic research. In Harrison, A., Clearwater, Y. A., and McKay, C. P. (Eds.). *From Antarctica to outer space: Life in isolation and confinement*. New York: Springer-Verlag, 1991, pp. 103–14.

146. Weybrew, B. B., and Alves, D. An exploratory study of the relationship of autonomic resiliency to manifest anxiety and selected personality traits. *U.S.N. Submarine Medical Research Laboratory Report No. 307*, 1959.

147. Weybrew B. B., Gessler, J. A., and Noddin, E. M. Factors related to drug abuse in the submarine service I. Selected demographic and psychometric data. *U.S.N. Submarine Medical Research Laboratory Report No. 726*, 1972.

148. Weybrew, B. B., and Jex, S. Stress in a seminar on stress: A methodological study. *Psychological Reports, 63, 1988*, 367–80.

149. Weybrew, B. B., and Molish, H. B. Attitude changes during and after long submarine missions. *Undersea Biomedical Research, 6, 1979*, 175–89.

150. Weybrew, B. B., and Molish, H. B. Prediction of nuclear submarine adaptability

from autonomic indices and Rorschach Inkblot responses. *U.S.N. Submarine Medical Research Laboratory Report No. 1080*, 1986.

151. Weybrew, B. B., Molish, H. B., and Youniss, R. P. Prediction of adjustment to the Antarctic. *U.S.N. Submarine Medical Research Laboratory Report No. 350*, 1961.
152. Weybrew, B. B., and Noddin, E. M. Factors related to the failure of enlisted submarine school graduates to qualify. *U.S.N. Submarine Medical Research Laboratory Report No. 586*, 1969.
153. Weybrew, B. B., and Noddin, E. M. Factors related to drug abuse in the submarine service II. Personality trait patterns as delineated by the Minnesota Multiphasic Personality Inventory (MMPI). *U.S.N. Submarine Medical Research Laboratory Report No. 737*, 1973.
154. Weybrew, B. B., and Noddin, E. M. Psychiatric aspects of the problem of adaptation to long submarine missions. *Aviation, Space, and Environmental Medicine, 50 (No. 6), 1979*, 575–80.
155. Weybrew, B. B., and Stark, J. E. Psychological and physiological changes associated with deprivation from smoking. *U.S.N. Submarine Medical Research Laboratory Report No. 490*, 1967.
156. Weybrew, B. B., and Youniss, R. P. The Personal Inventory Barometer (PIB): Development of the questionnaire. *U.S.N. Submarine Medical Research Laboratory Report No. 290*, 1957.
157. Wickramasekera, I. Electromyographic feedback training and tension headache: Preliminary observations. *American Journal of Clinical Hypnosis, 15, 1972*, 83.
158. Wilder, J. The law of initial value in neurology and psychiatry. *Journal of Nervous and Mental Disease, 125, 1957*, 73–86.
159. Wolpe, J. *Psychotherapy by reciprocal inhibition*. Palo Alto, CA: Stanford University Press, 1958.
160. Wolpe, J. *The practice of behavior therapy*. Oxford: Pergamon, 1969.
161. Wurtman, J. *Managing your mind and mood through food*. New York: Harper and Row, 1988.
162. Yalom, I. D. *The theory and practice of group psychotherapy*. New York: Basic Books, 1970.

Index

About the Author

BENJAMIN B. WEYBREW, Ph.D., received his doctorate in Clinical Psychology from the University of Colorado and is a recently retired Associate Professor from the University of New Haven. He was head of the Psychiatric Screening Branch of the U.S. Naval Submarine Research Laboratory, New London, Connecticut, from 1952–79, and has published many review articles and research papers dealing with stress and related topics.

www.ingramcontent.com/pod-product-compliance
Ingram Content Group UK Ltd.
Pitfield, Milton Keynes, MK11 3LW, UK
UKHW020810290926
15470UKWH00003B/1062

9 780275 942335